"This comprehensive resou[...] [...]c disease, including diagnosis an[...] [...]n entire chapter which contains invaluable advice from those with the most experience—people with celiac disease!"
    —Trisha B. Lyons, RD, LD, MetroHealth Medical Center, Cleveland, OH

"A clear and comprehensive guide for anyone newly diagnosed with celiac disease, complete with valuable resources."
    —Jessica Hale and Yvonne Gifford (*www.glutenfreeda.com*)

"An excellent resource for those dealing with celiac disease and also for those who care for people with the disease. An invaluable tool with loads of resources and useful information presented in a concise, easy-to-understand manner!"
    —Marla Doersch, RD

"A wonderfully comprehensive and invaluable guide to celiac disease, complete with the collective wisdom of the celiac community."
    —Bonnie J. Kruszka, author of *Eating Gluten-Free with Emily*

"This book is full of practical and helpful information on gluten-free living along with valuable tips and recipes from the experts themselves—those with celiac disease. This book would be a welcome addition to the celiac bookshelf!"
    —Shelley Case, BSc, RD, author of *Gluten-Free Diet: A Comprehensive Resource Guide*

Tell Me What to Eat If I Have Celiac Disease

Nutrition You Can Live With

By Kimberly A. Tessmer, RD, LD
Foreword by Elaine Magee

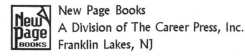

New Page Books
A Division of The Career Press, Inc.
Franklin Lakes, NJ

Tell Me What to Eat If I Have Celiac Disease
Edited by Diana Ghazzawi
Typeset by Gina Talucci
Cover design by Lucia Rossman, DigiDog Design
Printed in the U.S.A.

To order this title, please call toll-free 1-800-CAREER-1 (NJ and Canada: 201-848-0310) to order using VISA or MasterCard, or for further information on books from Career Press.

CAREER PRESS
New Page BOOKS

The Career Press, Inc., 3 Tice Road, PO Box 687,
Franklin Lakes, NJ 07417
www.careerpress.com
www.newpagebooks.com

Library of Congress Cataloging-in-Publication Data
Tessmer, Kimberly A.
    Tell me what to eat if I have celiac disease : nutrition you can live with / by Kimberly A. Tessmer.
        p. cm.
    Includes index.
    ISBN 978-1-60163-061-2
    1. Gluten-free diet. I. Title.

RM237.86.T474 2003
615.8'54--dc22

2008053975

Acknowledgments

This book is dedicated in loving memory to my mom, Nancy Bradford, who was my role model and taught me that anything is possible. She passed on to me her passion for helping others and has shown me the incredible strength people can have no matter what their circumstances. I thank her and my dad for all of the endless love and encouragement they have shown me throughout my life. I love you, Mom, and I miss you dearly!

Thank you to my entire family, especially my beautiful daughter, Tori, and my loving husband, Greg, for their constant love, support, and encouragement.

I sincerely thank all of the people who helped me in so many ways to write this book, including all of the people with celiac disease who shared their time, ideas, tips, stories, and recipes with the hope of helping others. A very special thank-you to Trisha Lyons, RD, LD; Kim Slominsky, RD, of Nutrition Evolution; and Regina Celano for your time and input into this book and for showing me the resilient, passionate, and caring spirit that people with celiac disease possess.

I give a huge thank-you to Shelley Case, RD, *the* gluten-free expert and the author of *Gluten-Free Diet: A Comprehensive Resource Guide* (Case Nutrition Consulting, 2008). You were such a valuable resource to me for this book; I appreciate your time and expertise. Thanks to Ann Whelan, editor and publisher of *Gluten-Free Living* magazine; Carol Fenster, PhD, of Savory Palate, Inc.; Jessica Hale, editor and chef of Glutenfreeda Online Cooking Magazine; Kenneth Fine, MD, of Intestinal Health Institute; Marla Doersch, RD; Bonnie Kruszka, author of *Eating Gluten-Free with Emily* (Woodbine House, 2004); Connie Sarros, author of *Wheat-Free, Gluten-Free Cookbook for Kids and Busy Adults* (McGraw-Hill, 2003); Bette Hagman, author of *The Gluten-Free Gourmet Cooks Fast and Healthy* (Holt Paperbacks, 2000); Christine A. Krahling; Lindsay Amadeo; and Marcy Thorner of The Grammar Guru (*http://the-grammar-guru.com*).

Contents

Foreword

"Gluten-free" has fast become a nutrition buzzword in the past few years. Many want to know if they might be helped by eliminating gluten. There are people who absolutely need to follow a gluten-free diet due to the autoimmune disorder of the small intestine called celiac disease, and others who want to try it in the hope that it will improve the way they feel. Whatever your need or motivation, this book tells you everything you need to know about living the gluten-free way.

The grains that contain the protein gluten are pervasive in the American diet—namely the wheat, rye, and barley grains. The foods most often substituted for gluten-containing foods are potato, rice, corn and soy. Kimberly Tessmer takes you beyond these simple substitutions, giving information about celiac disease, other diseases and disorders linked with celiac disease, food labels, gluten-free kitchens, and gluten-free meals. You will find answers to questions such as:

- Should I avoid oats too?
- What other diseases and conditions are gluten-free diets sometimes used to treat?

- If I don't have the symptoms of celiac disease, how do I know if I have a less severe intolerance to gluten?
- Why do some people with celiac disease not experience the traditional symptoms?

While reading this book, I came across some surprising information. I learned that celiac disease can show up at any age and can sometimes be triggered by events like surgery, pregnancy, or childbirth, viral infections, or severe emotional stress. Another surprise was that celiac disease is one of the most misdiagnosed diseases in the United States today, often misdiagnosed as irritable bowel syndrome, colitis, Crohn's disease, diverticulitis, chronic fatigue syndrome, and others. Though I knew that the physical reaction to eating gluten could be immediate, I was surprised to learn it can be delayed for weeks in some people; no two reactions are alike when it comes to celiac disease.

Kimberly Tessmer gives practical advice and her kind voice is heard through the entire book. I am confident it will help improve the health of thousands of people who suffer from and struggle with celiac disease and gluten intolerance.

—Elaine Magee, MPH, RD
Nationally known as "The Recipe Doctor"
(*www.recipedoctor.com*) and author of *Tell Me What To Eat If I Have Irritable Bowel Syndrome*, *Tell Me What To Eat If I Have Acid Reflux*, and others in the *Tell Me What to Eat* series.

Introduction

Celiac disease has many names, such as *gluten intolerance*, *gluten-sensitive enteropathy*, and *non-tropical sprue*. Each name describes a lifelong autoimmune disorder in which a person's body cannot tolerate a group of grain proteins known collectively as gluten. Gluten can be found in wheat, rye, barley, and any derivatives of these grains. Celiac disease was once thought to be rare, but is slowly being recognized as one of the most prevalent genetic disorders in the United States.

The only definite treatment for celiac disease is strict adherence to a 100-percent gluten-free diet for life. Following a gluten-free diet is not an easy task, but it can help prevent complications and symptoms that are associated with this disease. People with celiac disease need help managing their diets and their lives and, through this book, I hope to provide enough practical information for them to do just that.

The good news is that individuals with celiac disease are not alone. There are all types of groups that provide resources and support for people with celiac disease and for their families. As awareness of this disease grows, so does the pool of resources. There are more choices today than ever before for people with celiac disease.

This book serves many purposes. It will help people who have been clinically diagnosed understand what celiac disease is and the complex diet therapy that treats it. It teaches those who have the disease (and their families) how to manage their diet so that they can lead a more comfortable, normal, and healthy life. Physicians, nurses, dietitians, chefs, food service staff, and other healthcare professionals may also find this source useful as they come in contact with people who suffer from celiac disease. This book also contains stories, tips, ideas, and recipes from people who have celiac disease. My hope is that people with celiac disease will feel more connected and inspired by others who share in their condition.

This book should not substitute visits to a physician and a dietitian who specializes in celiac disease and gluten-free diets. It should also not be used as your solitary means of treating your disease. Instead, the book should be used as a complement to their instruction and as a reference when needed.

Publisher's Note

At the time it was written, all information in this book was believed by the author to be correct and factual. Information on celiac disease and gluten-free food changes frequently, as research is ongoing. Always keep yourself up-to-date by reading current, reputable publications and continuing to check food ingredient lists. The author and the publisher disclaim any liability arising directly or indirectly from the use of this book. The author will not accept any responsibility for any omissions, misinterpretations, or misstatements that may exist within this book. The author does not endorse any product or company listed in this book. The author is not engaged in rendering medical services and this book should not be construed as medical advice, nor should it take the place of regular scheduled appointments with your physician and/ or dietitian. Please, consult your healthcare professional for medical advice.

Chapter 1

Everything You Ever Wanted to Ask About Celiac Disease

There are plenty of questions that will come up if you or a family member is diagnosed with celiac disease. Following are some of the most common questions and their much needed answers. If you have questions, never be afraid to ask your doctor and dietitian to get the answers you need!

Q: What is celiac disease?

Celiac disease is an autoimmune disorder of the small intestines that can surface at any age. People with celiac disease must avoid all foods that contain gluten, which is found in wheat, rye, barley, and their derivatives. For people with celiac disease, consuming gluten causes an autoimmune reaction that triggers the destruction of the villi within the inner lining of the small intestines. Their bodies produce antibodies that attack the small intestines, causing damage and illness.

The destruction of the villi of the small intestines results in the body's inability to absorb nutrients that are needed for good health, such as carbohydrates, protein, fat, vitamins, and minerals. These nutritional deficiencies can deprive the brain, nervous system, bones, liver, heart, and other organs of the nourishment they need and can cause vitamin and mineral deficiencies, leading to many types of illnesses. Celiac disease is not curable, and there are currently no medications to treat it. The only form of treatment is strict adherence to a 100-percent gluten-free diet for life. Once on a gluten-free diet, symptoms diminish and the small intestine begins to heal and return to normal.

Q: What is gluten?

Gluten is a general term used for the storage proteins, or prolamins, in wheat, rye, and barley. The names of the specific prolamins are gliadins, secalins, and hordeins, in wheat, rye, and barley, respectively. Gluten is the part of flour that gives dough its structure, provides leavening, and holds products together. The term *gluten-free* is used as a general reference to the diet for celiac disease and to describe a food or diet that is void of prolamins from wheat, rye, and barley.

Q: Is celiac disease basically a food allergy to gluten?

No, celiac disease is not a food allergy to gluten but an autoimmune disease. These are two different conditions and with each the body responds very differently to gluten.

Q: What are the symptoms of celiac disease?

Symptoms of celiac disease can vary widely between individuals, ranging from having no symptoms to suffering the most extreme symptoms. Both children and adults can experience one or more of the following symptoms:

- Reoccurring abdominal bloating and pain
- Pale and foul-smelling stool
- Depression

- Nausea and vomiting
- Bone or joint pain
- Diarrhea
- Muscle cramps
- Weight loss
- Constipation
- Iron deficiency with or without unexplained anemia
- Chronic alternating diarrhea with constipation
- Excessive flatulence
- Vitamin and mineral deficiencies
- Balance problems
- Migraines
- Edema or excessive fluid retention
- Seizures or other neurological reactions
- Chronic fatigue, weakness, and lack of energy
- Memory problems
- Lactose intolerance

Infants and children may also display these additional symptoms:
- Failure to grow and thrive
- Maturation problems
- Bloated abdomens
- Learning challenges and disabilities
- Behavioral changes, including irritability
- Dental enamel defects

As a result of the body's inability to absorb nutrients, people with celiac disease may also be affected by other health problems such as osteoporosis, anemia, muscle cramping, and fatigue. They may also experience arthritis, joint pain, reproductive difficulties, depression, and behavioral changes.

Many people with the disease are asymptomatic for years; it becomes active only after something, such as surgery, viral infection, severe emotional stress, pregnancy, or childbirth, triggers it. Research has discovered that symptoms of celiac disease not only appear in the gastrointestinal tract, but in the neurological, endocrine, orthopedic, reproductive, and hematological systems as well. It is essential to visit your physician if you have celiac disease symptoms for more than seven days or if you suspect that you have celiac disease at all.

Q: Do all people with celiac disease experience symptoms?

No. Some people with celiac disease may not show any symptoms. This is because they may have an undamaged part of their small intestines that is able to absorb enough nutrients to prevent experiencing some of these symptoms. However, even though they may not experience symptoms, they are still at risk for the complications and damage of celiac disease.

Q: How common is celiac disease?

New medical studies indicate that celiac disease is much more common than once thought. In fact, recent studies and advances in the technology of diagnosis show that more than 2 million Americans or about one out of every 133 people have celiac disease. The same research also indicated that celiac disease is twice as common as Crohn's disease, ulcerative colitis, and cystic fibrosis combined. The problem is that only one in 4,700 people are ever diagnosed. However, the rate at which adults are being diagnosed is increasing rapidly thanks to greater awareness and improved diagnostic skills.

This same research found that the presence of celiac disease in at-risk groups (people who either have celiac disease in the family or who have gastrointestinal symptoms) was one in 22 people in first-degree relatives, one in 39 people in second-degree relatives, and one in 56 people who had gastrointestinal symptoms or a disorder associated with celiac disease. Studies have also found a higher prevalence of celiac disease in people who have related health issues, such as type 1 diabetes, anemia, arthritis, osteoporosis, infertility, Turner Syndrome, and Down Syndrome, even if they do not show gastrointestinal symptoms.

Q: What is a gastroenterologist?

A gastroenterologist is a physician who specializes in the diagnosis and treatment of diseases and conditions of the digestive and intestinal system such as stomach pain, liver disease, diarrhea, IBS, ulcerative colitis, Crohn's disease, celiac disease, colon polyps, and cancer. They may further specialize in treating people in certain age groups such as pediatrics. Gastroenterologists can be certified by the Board of Internal Medicine, which is recognized by the American Board of Medical Specialties.

Q: How is celiac disease diagnosed?

If your physician suspects celiac disease, you should be referred to a gastroenterologist—a specialist in the areas of the stomach and intestines—who has expertise in celiac disease. Keep in mind that a gastroenterologist is not the only type of doctor who may notice symptoms. Other specialized doctors, such as endocrinologists, rheumatologists, OB/GYNs, dentists, and dermatologists, may also take part in observing signs and symptoms of celiac disease.

The first step in the diagnosis process is a blood screening test. Special types of blood antibody tests are used in screening for gluten intolerance. Tests may include either IgA tissue transglutaminase (TTG) or IgA endomysium (EMA), plus Total Serum IgA (to test for IgA deficiency). There are certain antibodies in the body that are produced by the immune system in response to substances that are perceived as threatening to the body. The amount of these particular antibodies is higher than normal in people with celiac disease who are consuming a diet that contains gluten. These antibody blood tests will show whether your system is responding negatively to gluten. If antibody blood tests come back positive, that indicates that a person needs further evaluation, specifically a biopsy. The blood antibody tests are not a definitive tool for diagnosing celiac disease. The absence of these antibodies does not guarantee a person does not have celiac disease, and the presence of them does not guarantee that a person has celiac disease.

If the blood tests, along with symptoms, suggest the probability of celiac disease, the next step would be a biopsy that would check for actual damage to the villi and confirm the results. A biopsy is the most conclusive test and the gold standard for diagnosing celiac disease. An intestinal biopsy involves a long, thin tube, called an endoscope, that is passed through the mouth and stomach and into the small intestines. The instrument is able to obtain a small sample of the villi, or tissue, of the small intestine. If damage to the villi is found, the physician may place the person on a gluten-free diet for at least six months and then perform a second biopsy, to see if the lining has healed. Because celiac disease can cause malnutrition, tests are also done to help evaluate the person's nutritional status. Procedures will differ depending on your physician, but most physicians will accept a positive antibody test, one positive biopsy, and improvement of symptoms after a gluten-free diet as sufficient evidence for a positive diagnosis of celiac disease. It should be noted that a person should *never* follow a gluten-free diet *before* having blood tests and/or a biopsy done, because this can interfere with test results and lead to an incorrect diagnosis.

To recap, a proper diagnosis for celiac disease will include the following steps:

1. A suspicion of celiac disease based on symptoms, physical appearance, and abnormal antibody blood tests.
2. A small intestinal biopsy that shows damage to the villi.
3. Definite improvement with a total gluten-free diet.

Americans are not routinely screened or tested for the antibodies to gluten. However, because celiac disease is genetic, family members (especially immediate family of people who have been diagnosed) should be screened for the disease. That includes people who are asymptomatic. The longer a person with celiac disease goes undiagnosed and untreated, the greater his or her chances are of developing severe malnutrition and other health complications. It is also suggested that people who have other autoimmune disorders be screened for celiac disease.

Q: Can I eat any amount of gluten?

No. Once on a gluten-free diet, a person with celiac disease must follow a strict 100-percent gluten-free diet. Any amount of gluten in the diet can begin to cause damage to the small intestines, even if it does not cause symptoms.

Q: Is there a cure for celiac disease?

No, there is currently no cure or drug that will treat celiac disease. However, possibilities are continually being researched. Fortunately, people with celiac disease can lead a perfectly normal and healthy life by following a strict gluten-free diet. Some people may require additional medical therapy for other health issues caused and/or related to celiac disease.

Q: Is celiac disease genetic?

Yes, genetic factors are involved with celiac disease. It is still unclear whether a dominant or a recessive gene passes on the disease. Research shows that members of the immediate family of a person with celiac disease have about a 5- to 15-percent chance of developing the disease.

Q: How is celiac disease treated?

A strict, 100-percent gluten-free diet for life is the only known treatment for celiac disease. Following a gluten-free diet means avoiding any food products and beverages that contain wheat, rye, barley, and their derivatives. This means avoiding most starches, pasta, cereal, breads, and many processed foods that contain those grains. Once gluten is removed from the diet, the villi and tissues of the small intestine can begin to heal, and associated symptoms will begin to diminish. The National Digestive Disease's Information Clearinghouse (NDDIC), a service of the National Institute of Diabetes and Digestive and Kidney Diseases (NIDDK), states on its Website (*www2.niddk.nih.gov*), "For most people, following this diet will stop symptoms, heal existing intestinal damage, and prevent further damage. Improvement begins within days of starting the diet. The small intestine usually heals in three to six months in children but may take several years in adults. A healed intestine means a person now has villi that can absorb nutrients from food into the bloodstream."

A gluten-free diet must be followed for a lifetime, not just until the intestines are healed. Eating any amount of gluten can cause tissue damage, whether there are symptoms present or not. During the first few months of the gluten-free diet, or until the villi of the small intestines has healed, your physician may supplement your diet with vitamins and minerals to remedy any deficiencies and to replenish your body's nutrient stores. If lactose intolerance has developed, a lactose-free diet will also be necessary, though this often returns to normal within a few months of starting a gluten-free diet.

The diet of a person with celiac disease can be healthy, tasty, and well-balanced. It is vital to learn how to read food labels, become familiar with ingredients, and substitute foods that contain gluten with foods such as potato, rice, corn, and soy. Although adhering to a strict gluten-free diet can be challenging at times, it is becoming easier as more gluten-free products become available at your neighborhood supermarket. A gluten-free diet can be a complicated one, and a person on a gluten-free diet must be extremely vigilant when eating at home, eating at restaurants, buying lunch at school or work, eating at parties, or grabbing food from a vending machine. With the right education and with enough practice, living with a gluten-free diet can become second nature. It is vital to have the right attitude! Accept your disease, educate yourself, and move on. Don't let the disease control your life! Instead, control the disease and live a normal, healthy, happy life. Seek professional guidance from an experienced dietitian to help you get started in the right direction.

The most important aspects of treatment for a celiac-disease sufferer involves:

- Maintaining strict adherence to a gluten-free diet for life.

- Learning how to self-manage your diet.

- Helping others in your life to understand the basics of a gluten-free diet.

- Adapting the diet to fit it into everyday life and making any adjustments necessary for other special needs beyond that.

- Adjusting for other potential needs related to blood test evaluations that include levels of vitamins and minerals.

- Evaluating bone mineral density with the appropriate follow-ups as indicated by your physician.

- Continuous monitoring by your physician to evaluate your progress, medical status, and any changes in your condition that may call for additional treatment.

Q: What are the complications associated with celiac disease?

If left untreated, celiac disease can be life-threatening. People with celiac disease are likely to be afflicted with health problems that are related to malabsorption (the inability to absorb nutrients into the body), including osteoporosis, osteopenia, tooth enamel defects, pancreatic disease, central and peripheral nervous system disease, internal hemorrhaging, organ disorders (gallbladder, liver, or spleen), and gynecological disorders. People who do not adhere strictly to a gluten-free diet stand a greater risk of developing certain types of cancer (lymphoma and adencarcinoma) of the intestines. Some of the complications that accompany celiac disease can be healed or the risk lowered after adequate time on a gluten-free diet.

Q: Is celiac disease ever misdiagnosed as another illness or disease?

Yes. Celiac disease can be very difficult to diagnose, because its symptoms mirror those of other gastrointestinal disorders, such as irritable bowel syndrome (IBS), Crohn's disease, ulcerative colitis, diverticulosis, and intestinal infections; chronic fatigue syndrome; and depression. The average length of time from the start of symptoms and a confirmed diagnosis in the United States is currently 11 years. If your physician suspects celiac disease you should be referred to a gastroenterologist (a specialist in the areas of the stomach and intestines) who has experience with celiac disease.

Q: What is lactose intolerance, and how is it related to celiac disease?

Lactose is a natural sugar found in milk and milk products. Lactose intolerance is a condition that stems from a deficiency of lactase, the enzyme that is needed to break down lactose. Symptoms of lactose intolerance may include some or all of the following: bloating, gas, abdominal cramping, diarrhea, nausea, and headache. For people with celiac disease, lactose intolerance is more prevalent, because the damage to the gastrointestinal tract can reduce the level of lactase in the body. Lactose intolerance is usually only temporary until the condition is under control and the small intestine heals.

Q: Is there a connection between celiac disease and diabetes?

Yes. There is a strong correlation between celiac disease and type 1 diabetes. The prevalence of type 1 diabetes in the general population is about 0.5 percent where in people with celiac disease it is approximately five to 10 percent. There has been no connection found between celiac disease and the more common form of type 2 diabetes.

Q: What is dermatitis herpetiformis, and what does it have to do with gluten?

Dermatitis herpetiformis (DH) is a chronic and severe disease of the skin that causes itchy skin blisters on the elbows, knees, buttocks, scalp, and back. DH is also a genetic autoimmune disease and is linked to celiac disease. In fact, about five percent of people with celiac disease will develop DH, either before being diagnosed or within the first year on the diet. Like celiac disease, DH is also treated with a gluten-free diet as well as medications to control the skin rash.

Most people with DH do not have obvious gastrointestinal symptoms, but almost all will show some type of damage to the small intestines. Therefore, they too have the potential for all of the nutritional problems and damage of a person with celiac disease. Both celiac disease and DH are permanent, and symptoms and damage will occur if gluten is consumed.

Q: What other diseases or disorders are linked with celiac disease?

There seems to be a higher occurrence of other diseases and disorders, many of them other autoimmune disorders, for people with celiac disease. The connection between celiac disease and some of these diseases or disorders may be strictly genetic. Some of these diseases and disorders include:

- Dermatitis herpetiformis (DH)
- Kidney disease
- Insulin-dependent type 1 diabetes
- Carcinoma of the oropharynx, esophagus, and small bowel
- Thyroid disease
- Liver disease
- Sjogrens syndrome
- Graves' disease
- Systemic lupus erythematosus
- Addison's disease
- Rheumatoid arthritis
- Chronic active hepatitis
- IgA nephropathy and IgA deficiency
- Scleroderma
- Down syndrome

Most recently it has been reported that a gluten-free diet may help other conditions such as autism, chronic fatigue syndrome, multiple sclerosis, and attention-deficit hyperactivity disorder. These findings are not yet proven, but more research is currently being conducted. A gluten-free diet is not, by any means, a cure for any of these conditions, but it could offer relief of symptoms for some. Talk to your healthcare provider about the possible benefits of a gluten-free diet for you. Knowing that people with celiac disease have a greater incidence of certain health problems, emphasis should be put on visiting your physician for regular check-ups and taking care of your health.

Q: Is there a link between autism and gluten-free diets?

Some groups are now advocating protocol that recognizes prescribing a gluten-free, casein-free (free of a protein fraction found in dairy products) diet for at least three months to children who show autistic behavior. It may take at least a three-month trial period to actually determine if the diet makes a difference. There has recently been a growing body of research that shows that the inability to break down certain foods (such as the proteins in gluten and casein) may affect the developing brain in some children, causing some autistic behavior. These undigested, unbroken proteins (called peptides) are normally excreted in the urine, though a few enter the bloodstream. Unbroken peptides that enter the bloodstream attach to the opiate receptors of the child's brain and seem to cause abnormal brain development and an opiate-like effect. (Opiates are highly addictive and can reach toxic levels.) The opiate-like effect can cause the child to feel drowsy, block pain receptors, and depress the activity of the nervous system. A urine test can detect unbroken peptides. If high levels of the unbroken peptides show up in the urine, it may be worth placing the child on a gluten-free, casein-free diet. Research has not yet proven that a gluten-free, casein-free diet will help every child with autistic behaviors, but it is still being carried out. For more information, research the Websites of the Autism Society of America (*http:/ /www.autism-society.org*) and the Autism Network for Dietary Intervention (*http://www.autismndi.com*).

Q: How do I communicate with my physician?

Your first order of business is to find a physician who meets your special needs. Depending on your healthcare plan, you may need to be referred to a specialist, usually a gastroenterologist, by your primary care provider. Your physician should be someone you completely trust and with whom you feel comfortable speaking to about concerns, suspicions, and feelings. Your physician should be someone who is open to any new information you have learned concerning celiac disease. Find a physician who allows you to actively participate in your own healthcare and who provides any support and assistance necessary to diagnose and treat your disease. Be sure that the physician you choose has adequate knowledge of celiac disease and is willing to screen patients for this particular disease.

It is a smart idea to keep copies of all your medical records, to which you are legally entitled. This keeps you more in control and up-to-date with your disease and treatment, and it will also make it easier if you need to change doctors at any point. Be sure to schedule an exam every year, along with any tests that are appropriate for your age and risk factors. It is important for people with celiac disease to have a gluten antibody test once a year to monitor their response to their gluten-free diet. A positive test would let you know that you need to follow your gluten-free diet a bit closer. Other annual screenings should include thyroid and blood tests to measure for folic acid, calcium, iron, and vitamins D, A, K, and B12. Bone density should also be tested annually for individuals who have abnormal results.

When choosing a specialist, you can begin by consulting your primary care provider. A second information source could be your local county's medical societies. Another excellent route is to contact the state university medical center in your area. You can call and ask for a referral or a phone number for the chair of the department of gastroenterology. A state university medical center will make other specialty departments more accessible to you in case you need them, as well as provide you with a substantial medical team to monitor all aspects of your condition.

Q: What questions should I ask my physician?

It is important to be prepared before you visit your doctor. Know what questions you plan to ask ahead of time and write them down so you won't forget them. If you suspect you have celiac disease, do your homework and brush up on the basics before your visit. During your visit, ask whatever questions you feel you need answers to and don't be intimidated! This is your health and your body; you have the right to know and understand what is going on. Write down the answers to your questions and, if the doctor is not clear with an answer, ask him to clarify it. Repeat the doctor's answers to verify that you understand. Be sure to let the doctor know if there are others in your family who have celiac disease or who are experiencing the same type of symptoms that you are. If possible, bring a friend or family member along with you. Sometimes it helps to have at least two pairs of ears listening for better understanding and retention.

Don't be rushed out of the doctor's office. Stay until you feel all of your questions have been answered and you fully understand your condition, diagnosis, treatment, and so forth. Before you leave the doctor's office make sure you know exactly how to contact the doctor for any follow-up questions that may arise. Most importantly, if you are not getting the results you want from your doctor or specialist, seek the advice of another physician. You have every right to get to the bottom of your symptoms and improve your health. Just because a physician is a gastroenterologist does not necessarily mean he or she specializes in celiac disease, so you may have to consult more than one specialist.

The following are some important questions to ask your physician, whether you suspect you may have celiac disease or if you have been diagnosed with celiac disease and are searching for a physician:

- What is your background and experience with celiac disease?
- How many patients with celiac disease have you seen in the last year?
- How rare or common is celiac disease?
- What causes celiac disease?
- Can you explain celiac disease and its symptoms?
- How is celiac disease diagnosed?
- How is celiac disease treated?
- Should my family members be screened for celiac disease if I have it?
- Is it okay to have some gluten in the diet?
- Should I take vitamin or mineral supplements?
- Could I have associated food intolerances?
- Why and where should I have a bone density test done?
- What other tests should I have done now and on a regular basis?
- What concerns should I have from celiac disease?
- What complications could I experience with celiac disease?
- Who can best teach me about a gluten-free diet?

Q: What can help me live more easily with celiac disease?

Living with celiac disease can be very challenging. However, as you learn more, managing your disease will become second nature. Use the following suggestions to help you cope more easily as you begin following your diet:

Collect all the information you can about celiac disease and gluten-free diets. Talk to your physician, search the Internet (make sure to stick with reputable Websites), read books and pamphlets, purchase specialized gluten-free cookbooks, and become familiar with gluten-free associations and groups. Knowledge is power. The more you know, the more control you have and the easier life with celiac disease will become. As you learn, educate your loved ones. It is just as important for your family members to understand the basics of a gluten-free diet.

Don't go it alone! Seek out others who have celiac disease and can help and support you through the tough times. There are plenty of local support groups, as well as chat rooms and message boards, on the Internet that can help provide all kinds of support.

Be sure to seek the guidance of a professional. Getting started can be difficult and overwhelming, so don't hesitate to speak to a registered dietitian who specializes in celiac disease and gluten-free diets. A dietitian can help you sort through the foods you are allowed and not allowed, as well as provide you with valuable information. You can search the American Dietetic Association's Website (*www.eatright.org*) to find a dietitian in your area, or ask your physician to refer you to one. Keep in mind that you should choose a dietitian and physician who specialize in celiac disease and gluten-free diets.

Chapter 2

All About Gluten-Free Diets

We have already established that the only treatment for people with celiac disease is a lifelong adherence to a gluten-free eating regimen and that there are also other health conditions, such as dermatitis herpetiformis, that require a gluten-free (GF) diet for life. What follows are some frequently asked questions about gluten-free diets and their answers.

Q: Who needs to follow a gluten-free diet?

For people with celiac disease, eating any food that contains gluten, a protein found in wheat, rye, barley, and any derivative of these grains, sets off an autoimmune response that causes the destruction of the villi within the lining of the small intestines, as well as the destruction of digestive enzymes. Their body produces antibodies that attack the small intestines, causing damage, illness, and, in most, severe symptoms.

In addition to celiac disease, gluten-free diets are also used to treat dermatitis herpetiformis (DH). DH is a chronic and severe skin disease that causes itchy skin blisters on the elbows, knees, buttocks, scalp, and back. When a person with DH consumes gluten, it triggers an immune system response that deposits a substance, immunoglobulin gamma A (IgA), under the top layer of the skin. Once the IgA is deposited under the skin, a gluten-free diet can slowly clear it but it takes time. Most people with DH do not have obvious gastrointestinal symptoms, but almost all have some type of damage to the small intestines. Therefore, they too have the potential for all of the nutritional problems of a person with celiac disease, including malnutrition and malabsorption. Both celiac disease and DH are life-long conditions. With both, symptoms and damage will occur if gluten is consumed. A strict gluten-free diet needs to be followed for life. Treatment for DH may also include certain drugs that can dramatically relieve the burning, itching, and rash on the skin.

There are also people who suffer from a less aggressive form of gluten intolerance. This is even harder to diagnose than celiac disease, because there are no established diagnostic criterion. People who may have a general intolerance to gluten do not experience the severe symptoms that those who have celiac disease experience, but a gluten-free diet can substantially improve their health and quality of life.

Q: Is a gluten-free diet healthy?

Following a gluten-free diet should not mean that you can no longer follow a healthy diet. Your main focus should still be to eat well-balanced meals and to eat from all of the food groups each day. The key is to build your healthy eating plan using alternative grains.

Foods with whole wheat flours, such as breads, cereals, and pastas, are great sources of complex carbohydrates, fiber, and nutrients such as B vitamins and iron. In the United States, most refined wheat flours, wheat-based food products, and cereals are enriched with thiamin, riboflavin, niacin, folic acid, and iron. Unfortunately, those with celiac disease cannot eat any of these foods, and many of the gluten-free grain products are not enriched.

Therefore, many of the specially made gluten-free grain products may not provide the same amount of nutrients as their wheat-containing counterparts.

Another essential dietary element to consider is fiber, because wheat is a large contributor of dietary fiber in an average diet, and because many gluten-free foods are low in fiber. Therefore, it is important to ensure that you consume the recommended amount of fiber daily. The chart below shows the recommended daily intake of fiber.

U.S. Food and Nutrition Board Fiber Recommendations

Men younger than 50 years	38 grams daily
Women younger than 50 years	25 grams daily
Men older than 50 years	30 grams daily
Women older than 50 years	21 grams daily

In order increase your intake of B vitamins, iron, and fiber:

- Eat a variety of fresh fruits and vegetables daily (at least five servings or more per day).
- Include other high-fiber, gluten-free foods daily, such as legumes (dried beans), nuts, and seeds.
- Eat the edible skins of fruits and vegetables, such as those of apples and potatoes. The skin contains most of the fiber in some produce.
- Choose whole-grain gluten-free products as opposed to refined, gluten-free grains. For example, use brown rice instead of white rice.
- Choose gluten-free products that incorporate higher nutritive gluten-free grains, such as buckwheat, bean, quinoa, amaranth, and soy.
- Couple foods that are high in vitamin C with iron-rich foods to increase your absorption of iron.
- Drink coffee or tea between meals, instead of with meals, to ensure iron is being absorbed to its fullest.

- Increase your intake of foods that are naturally gluten-free and are higher in the B vitamins and iron, such as lean meats, legumes, eggs, peanut butter, fish, most dairy products, green leafy vegetables, brown rice, nuts (almonds), seeds (sunflower), fruit juices (orange and tomato), potatoes, and basically all other plant foods.

- Talk to your doctor about taking a daily gluten-free multi-vitamin/mineral supplement, as well as a gluten-free calcium supplement. If you are not sure how much to take or what brand to use, contact your dietitian or physician.

Q: Can I eat oats?

The use of oats in a gluten-free diet has been an ongoing controversy, because their safety was questioned. The problem in the past with including oats on a gluten-free diet was that, even if the oats themselves were a safe grain, there was always the concern of cross-contamination from grains that contained gluten. Current research is finding that eating pure, uncontaminated oats, in moderation, is safe for most people with celiac disease. However, some people with celiac disease show sensitivity to oats, whether pure or not. Ideally, if a person wants to include oats in their gluten-free diet, they need to consume only those oat products that have been tested and found to be pure and free of contamination.

According to their Website (*www.gluten.net*), the Gluten Intolerance Group of North America's (GIG) position on the matter states, "Research shows that pure, uncontaminated oats in moderation (1/2 cup dry daily) are safe for most persons with celiac disease. Because it remains questionable whether all people with celiac disease can tolerate oats, it is advised that they work closely with their healthcare team before adding oats to their daily diet and that they have their antibody levels checked periodically to assure the addition of oats is not causing any damage."

Q: How do I get my gluten-free diet started?

Keep in mind that adjusting to anything new takes time. Don't expect to learn everything you need to know overnight. It is very normal to feel overwhelmed and upset about favorite foods that you must now avoid. However, there is a large variety of gluten-free foods available, and that number will continue to increase as the number of people that are diagnosed with celiac disease increases.

Your first important step is education. You must read labels before you eat any food and become skilled at doing so. If the food contains an ingredient that is questionable, then avoid the food until you can learn more about it. While you are learning about all the foods you can or cannot eat, try to stick with foods that are naturally gluten-free, such as plain poultry, fish, and meats; legumes; plain potatoes and rice; and fresh fruits and vegetables. Most dairy products can also be consumed as long as you are not lactose intolerant. All of these foods are healthy and delicious! The key is being careful to prepare these foods without other gluten-containing products.

Use some of these helpful tips to get your gluten-free diet started:

- Learn to focus on foods you can eat instead of foods that you cannot eat.
- Learn everything you can about gluten-free foods and keep notes for yourself on what you have learned. Keep a list of "safe" foods to act as a quick reference.
- If you have questions about a certain food, go right to the source and contact the manufacturer.
- Keep a food diary to help you become more familiar with gluten-free foods and meals. Take notes about foods you have investigated and write down what you eat and how your body reacts. This may also give you a clue about patterns that indicate other food sensitivities.

- When in doubt, do without! Don't eat anything that is questionable.

- Because many people who are newly diagnosed with celiac disease are lactose intolerant, you may want to wait two to four months to introduce dairy products into your diet. After the intestine heals, people with celiac disease who were not lactose intolerant before developing celiac disease will usually return to being able to tolerate lactose.

- Don't rely on your body's response to gauge whether you can eat a food or not. If a food contains gluten, it should not be a part of your diet, whether it causes symptoms or not. Some people may not experience symptoms when consuming small amounts of gluten, but damage to the small intestines continues.

- Get into the habit of reading foods labels on all prepared and/or processed foods before you buy them and consume them. Many manufacturers reformulate their products on a regular basis, so labels should be checked frequently. Learn all the ingredients that include gluten as "hidden" component.

- Be careful to choose "gluten-free foods," as opposed to "gluten-restricted foods," unless you are absolutely positive it does not contain gluten.

- Be aware that just because a food is "wheat-free," does not mean it is "gluten-free."

- Watch for cross-contamination between utensils, toasters, counters, food storage bins, jars, and any other place people may leave crumbs.

- Be careful of taking advice from employees at places such as health-food stores. Go right to a professional for reliable help.

- When dining out, don't be afraid to speak up and ask questions about how food is prepared or to ask to have something specially prepared for you.

- Don't let grocery shopping confuse you. Remember that the perimeter of the store is where the fresh foods are usually located. Many stores now have special sections where they often stock gluten-free foods. Ask if you cannot find them.

- Visit health-food or organic stores in your area to look for gluten-free foods that will complement your daily meal plans. It's wise to visit several stores, because each one may stock different types of food. Talk to the staff about ordering special foods that you want if you cannot find them at the store.

- A large variety of gluten-free products are available through mail order or on Websites.

- Join a support group. It is invaluable to have other people that you can lean on for support.

- Invest in some good gluten-free cookbooks and start your own library. Swap recipes with friends you meet in support groups.

- Contact a dietitian who specializes in celiac disease to help you get started on the right path. They will have the answers you need.

- Be prepared for events such as hospital stays. Be sure to speak to the staff dietitian in advance concerning your special dietary needs. Also, ask that the kitchen and nursing staffs be notified. If you don't feel the hospital will be able to accommodate your gluten-free needs, have someone bring you food from home. Be sure you clear the situation with your physician or staff nurse and that your specific orders are included on your medical chart.

- Carry small treats for yourself, tucked in your pocket or purse. Following a gluten-free diet does not mean you can't have scrumptious treats when at the movies or the ballpark!

Q: What should I ask manufacturers?

If you can't decipher whether a food contains gluten by reading a food label, then it is best to go right to the source and contact the manufacturer. You should be able to find the address, phone number, or Website listed on the package. Before you call or e-mail the manufacturer, be sure you know what to ask and be specific about what you are asking. It is a smart idea to ask the customer representative at the company to reflect the question you asked in his or her answer so that you can be sure that he or she understood your question and is answering it correctly.

Calling the manufacturer will increase your chances of an immediate response. Have the label in front of you when calling and ask the customer representative specific questions about specific ingredients. Instead of asking if a product is gluten-free, ask about the sources of specific ingredients such as wheat, barley, rye, modified food starch, or flavorings. It is also important to question contamination issues, even if the food is gluten-free. Ask if equipment is cleaned between batches or if separate equipment is used for the gluten-free products. Finally, keep a list of the phone numbers, Websites, and e-mail addresses that you use so that you can check back frequently or investigate new products.

Q: What should I look for on food labels?

The importance of reading food labels before buying or consuming foods cannot be stressed enough. There are foods with obvious sources of gluten, but many more have much less apparent sources. There are many ingredients that have alternate or "hidden" names, as well as derivatives from gluten-containing grains, that are used during production.

The Food Allergen Labeling and Consumer Protection Act (FALCPA) took effect in January of 2006. It requires food labels to now clearly identify wheat and other common food allergens, eight in total, on a food product's list of ingredients. The problem for people following a gluten-free diet is that barley, rye, and oats are not included in this allergen-labeling law. Therefore, it is still necessary check with companies to determine whether a food product is indeed gluten-free. There are many manufacturers that have voluntarily chosen to list all gluten ingredients and others who are now adding the words "gluten-free" to appropriate food labels. If a Kraft Food product, for example, contains any type of gluten (which, for labeling purposes, includes wheat, rye, barley, and oats) the source of gluten will be listed on the ingredient list, no matter how small the amount may be.

Recently proposed requirements now require food companies to meet new standards before labeling their food products as "gluten-free". For the first time the Food and Drug Administration (FDA) has proposed defining the term gluten-free. This helps give people with celiac disease greater confidence that specially labeled foods are in fact safe to eat. According to their Website (*www.fda.gov*), the FDA proposal defines the term "gluten-free" to mean that a food being labeled or claiming it is "gluten-free" does NOT contain any one of the following:

- An ingredient that is a prohibited grain.
- An ingredient that is derived from a prohibited grain and that has not been processed to remove gluten.
- An ingredient that is derived from a prohibited grain and that has been processed to remove gluten, if the use of that ingredient results in the presence of 20 ppm (parts per million) or more gluten in the food.
- 20 ppm or more gluten.

Q: What ingredients should I avoid on a gluten-free diet?

There are many of the ingredients to avoid on a gluten-free diet. Some of the most common are in the following list, which is part of the more inclusive one found on the Celiac.com Website (*www.celiac.com*). Since this is not an all-inclusive list, you should question all ingredients that you are not sure about. Avoid foods that list these ingredients on their labels:

- All-purpose or enriched flour (unless labeled GF)
- Barley, barley malt, barley grass
- Beer (unless GF), ale, stout, porter, and any other similar fermented beverages
- Bleached flour
- Bran
- Bread flour
- Bromated flour
- Bulgur
- Cereal extract and binding
- Couscous
- Cracked wheat
- Cracker meal
- Durum/durum flour
- Einkorn
- Emmer
- Farina
- Filler
- Flour (It is normally wheat-based.)
- Graham flour
- Groats (wheat, barley)
- Hydrolyzed wheat gluten

- Hydrolyzed wheat protein
- Hydrolyzed wheat starch
- Kamut
- Malt
- Malt beverages or malted milk
- Malt extract
- Malt flavoring (It is often used in cereals.)
- Malt syrup
- Malt vinegar
- Mir
- Pearl barley
- Phosphated flour
- Rice malt
- Ryc
- Seitan
- Self-rising flour
- Semolina
- Spelt
- Triticale
- Wheat
- Wheat bran
- Wheat germ
- Wheat grass
- Wheat starch (It is wheat with the gluten washed out, but it is not considered gluten-free.)
- Whole meal flour

The items in the previous list, some which have "hidden" names, indicate the presence of some type of gluten grain on a food label and should be avoided on a gluten-free diet.

Q: Are there any other ingredients that may contain gluten that a person with celiac disease should avoid?

There are some food ingredients that may or may not be made from grains that may be toxic to the person with celiac disease.

According to the U.S. Code of Federal Regulations by FDA (*www.fda.gov*), dextrin is an incompletely hydrolyzed starch and is an ingredient that is used as a thickening agent, binder, and diluting agent for pills and capsules. It can also be found in baked goods, candy, gravies, pie fillings, poultry, puddings, soups, supplements, and medications. According to FDA regulations, dextrin can be produced from corn, waxy maize, waxy milo, potato, arrowroot, rice, tapioca, sago, or wheat starches. Most dextrin used in the United States is made from corn or tapioca. However, people on a gluten-free diet should be in the habit of always checking the source when this ingredient appears on a label. Maltodextrin, when listed as an ingredient on foods sold in the United States, must be made from corn or potato per FDA regulations.

Caramel coloring is an ingredient used to color foods. It is produced by the careful heat treatment of certain carbohydrates, either alone or in the presence of food-grade acids, alkalis, and salts. The following carbohydrates can be used: dextrose, invert sugar, lactose, malt syrup, molasses, starch hydrolysates, and sucrose. Corn is used most often in the United States, because it has a longer shelf life and produces a better food product. If made outside the United States, it could possibly contain gluten.

Hydrolyzed vegetable protein/hydrolyzed plant protein (HVP/HPP) is an ingredient that is used as a flavor enhancer in many processed foods such as soups, chili, sauces, stews, and some meat products, such as hot dogs. A specific protein (such as soy, corn, or wheat) is broken down into amino acids by a chemical process called hydrolysis. The terms HVP and HPP are no longer allowed to be used on U.S. food labels. The source of the protein must now be stated. The U.S. Code of Federal Regulations by the FDA states, "The common or usual name of a protein hydrolysate shall be specific to the ingredient and shall include the identity of the food source from which the protein was derived. 'Hydrolyzed wheat gluten,' 'hydrolyzed soy protein,' and 'autolyzed yeast extract' are examples of acceptable names. 'Hydrolyzed casein' is also an example of an acceptable name, whereas 'hydrolyzed milk protein' is not acceptable because it is not specific to the ingredient (hydrolysates can be prepared from other milk proteins). The names 'hydrolyzed vegetable protein' and 'hydrolyzed protein' are not acceptable, because they do not identify the food source of the protein."

The FDA's U.S. Code of Federal Regulations also states that modified food starch can be produced from corn, tapioca, potato, wheat, or other starches. It is gluten-free unless it is made from wheat. If modified food starch is made from wheat, then "wheat" will appear on the food label. Presently, the FDA does not require that the identity of the modified food starch be revealed on food labels. According to FDA regulations, when the word starch appears on its own as an ingredient, it is considered cornstarch. If it is any other type of starch the ingredient must designate what type of starch it is, such as "wheat starch." There is no standard such as this for modified food starch, so it must be questioned when found on food labels.

"Artificial and natural flavorings," as they are often termed on ingredient lists, can be made from a variety of grains, including wheat, rye, and barley. Most U.S. manufactures do not use gluten-containing flavorings, but there are a few exceptions. Barley malt is sometimes used as a flavoring and some companies may not always declare it as a flavor containing barley. Hydrolyzed wheat, corn, and/or soy protein can be used as a flavor or flavor enhancer in all types of foods.

Because manufactures tend to change formulations quite often, check the labels of these foods on a regular basis. Foods should not be consumed unless you have verified that they contain none of the prohibited grains. Though this is not an all inclusive list, you should question all of the following foods and ingredients:

- Bullion cubes
- Brown rice syrup
- Candy
- Cold cuts
- Communion wafers
- Emulsifier
- Flavorings in meat
- French fries (At restaurants, check if they are fried in a fryer that is used for other foods.)
- Gelatinized or pre-gelatinized starch
- Gravies
- Hot dogs
- Imitation bacon
- Imitation pepper
- Imitation seafood
- Mono- and diglycerides (in dry products only)
- Rice mixes
- Sauces
- Sausage
- Seasonings (unspecified)
- Seasoned snacks, such as tortilla chips and potato chips
- Self-basting turkey
- Soups
- Soy sauce (Check label to make sure it is wheat-free.)

- Stabilizers
- Textured vegetable protein (TVP)
- Thickeners
- Vegetables in sauce

Now that you have heard ingredients to avoid and question, here is a list of ingredients and additives that, according to Celiac.com (where you can find a more inclusive list), are gluten-free and are safe for the diet of a person with celiac disease:

- Acacia gum
- Adipic acid
- Agar
- Albumin
- Alfalfa
- Algin
- Aluminum
- Amaranth
- Amino acids
- Amylase
- Annatto/annatto color
- Arabic gum
- Arrowroot
- Ascorbic acid
- Aspartame
- Aspartic acid
- Baking yeast
- Bean flour
- Benzoic acid
- Beta-carotene
- BHA
- BHT
- Brewers yeast
- Buckwheat, pure
- Caffeine
- Calcium carbonate
- Calcium chloride
- Calcium disodium
- Calcium phosphate
- Calcium silicate
- Calcium stearate
- Calcium sulfate
- Canola oil
- Carboxymethyl cellulose
- Carob bean
- Carrageenan
- Casein
- Cellulose/cellulose gum

- Cetyl alcohol
- Citric acid
- Corn (bran, corn-starch, cornmeal, grits, hominy, corn gluten)
- Corn syrup/corn syrup solids
- Cream of tartar
- Demineralized whey
- Dextrose
- Dioctyl sodium
- Distilled vinegar (The single word "vinegar" on food labels in the United States denotes apple cider vinegar.)
- Ester gum
- Ethyl maltol
- Fava bean flour
- Flax seed
- Folic acid, folacin
- Fructose
- Fumaric acid
- Garbanzo flour
- Garfava flour
- Gelatin
- Glucose
- Glutamic acid
- Glutinous rice
- Glycerin/glycerol/glycerides
- Guar gum
- Gums (acacia, Arabic, carob bean, cellulose, guar, Karaya, locust bean, tragacanth, xanthan)
- Hydrochloric acid
- Invert sugar
- Karaya gum
- Kasha
- Keratin
- Lactase
- Lactic acid
- Lactose
- L-cysteine
- Lecithin
- Lipase
- Locust bean
- Lutein
- Magnesium hydroxide
- Maize
- Malic acid
- Maltodextrin
- Maltol/ethyl maltol
- Mannitol
- Methylcellulose
- Millet
- Mineral oil

- Molasses
- MSG (monosodium glutamate)
- Niacin/niacinamide
- Nitric acid
- Paprika
- Pectin
- Pepsin
- Phenylalanine
- Polyethylene glycol
- Polyglycerol
- Polysorbates 60 and 80
- Potassium citrate
- Potassium iodide
- Potassium sorbate
- Potato flour and/or starch
- Propylene glycol
- Psyllium
- Pyridoxine hydro-chloride
- Quinoa
- Riboflavin
- Rice (white, brown, wild)
- Rice bran
- Rice flour
- Sago
- Sodium benzoate
- Sodium caseinate
- Sodium citrate
- Sodium metabisulphite
- Sodium nitrate
- Sodium nitrate/ nitrate
- Sodium stearoyl lactylate
- Sorbitol-mannitol
- Sorghum
- Soy lecithin
- Splenda
- Stearamide
- Stearamine
- Stearates
- Stearic acid
- Sucralose
- Sucrose
- Sulfites
- Sulfur dioxide
- Tapioca flour
- Tartaric acid
- Tartrazine
- Teff
- Titanium dioxide
- Tragacanth gum
- Vanilla extract
- Vanilla flavoring
- Whey
- White sugar
- Xanthan gum
- Xylitol

Q: What are foods are allowed, not allowed, and questionable within common food groupings?

Plain poultry, fish, meats, legumes, potatoes, rice, fresh fruit, fresh vegetables, and most dairy products are naturally gluten-free and safe to eat. Rice, corn, soy, potato, tapioca, beans, sorghum, millet, buckwheat, quinoa, amaranth, arrowroot, teff, and nut flours are all safe to eat on a gluten-free diet. It is important to pay special attention to additives, stabilizers, thickeners, and preservatives, which may or may not contain gluten. Gluten is an obvious ingredient in many foods such as wheat products, breads, baked goods, cookies, cakes, and pasta. The difficulty still lies in the "hidden ingredients" in processed foods, candy, medications, seasonings, canned foods, salad dressings, and supplements that contain gluten. It is vital for people on gluten-free diets to learn how to recognize these hidden ingredients by reading food labels and asking questions. Check ingredient labels on foods listed as questionable before consuming.

The following lists, by food groups, categorize foods according to whether they are allowed, are questionable, or are not allowed. To "question" means that you should read the food label and check the ingredient list before consuming. The following lists have been adapted from *Gluten-Free Diet: A Comprehensive Resource Guide* (Case Nutrition Consulting, 2008) by Shelley Case, RD. They have also been reviewed by Kim Slominsky, RD, of Nutrition Evolution.

Dairy Products

Allowed: Milk (fat-free, 1-percent, 2-percent, or whole); cream; evaporated and condensed milk; butter milk; plain, unflavored yogurt; hard natural cheeses; cream cheese; processed cheese; cottage cheese.

To Question: Milk drinks or flavored milks; frozen yogurt; sour cream; processed cheese sauces and spreads; flavored cheeses; flavored or fruited yogurt; non-dairy creamers; ice cream; soy or rice milk.

To Avoid: Malted milk; ice cream made with unsafe ingredients.

Breads, Biscuits, Cereal, Crackers, and Grains

Allowed: Bread and baked goods made from safe flours such as rice (brown or white), corn (maize), soy, amaranth, arrowroot, pea, cornstarch, potato, whole bean, legume, tapioca, sago, rice bran, corn meal, millet, flax, teff, sorghum, taro/taro flour or quinoa; montina flour (good source of fiber); GF pure uncontaminated oats; GF breadcrumbs; pure corn taco shells; and pure corn tortillas.

Hot cereal: cream of rice; soy grits; hominy grits; cream of buckwheat; millet; cornmeal; quinoa flakes; rice flakes; amaranth cereals.

Cold cereal: puffed corn; puffed rice; puffed Millet; rice flakes; soy cereal; puffed buckwheat; amaranth cereal.

To Question: Buckwheat flour (pure buckwheat flour is gluten-free but it is sometimes mixed with wheat flour, so check ingredients); rice crackers; rice cakes; *all* cereals (even ones made with GF grains) should be checked for malt flavorings and/or malt extract.

To Avoid: Breads; baked products or cereals containing wheat, rye, triticale, barley, bulgur, wheat germ, wheat bran, wheat-based corn flour, graham flour, gluten flour, durum flour, wheat starch, oat bran, farina, wheat-based semolina, spelt, kamut, faro, German wheat/Dinkel, einkorn, enriched flour, and any other unsafe flour; cereals with added malt extract and malt flavoring; wheat flour tacos and tortillas; powdered mixes for waffles and pancakes.

Pasta and Rice

Allowed: Pasta, noodles or macaroni made from rice, corn, soy, quinoa, beans, potato and other allowed flours; rice (brown, white, wild); glutinous/sweet rice; kasha.

To Question: Soba/Buckwheat pasta; boxed rice mixes.

To Avoid: Any type of pasta made from wheat, wheat starch, or any other flour/grain not allowed; couscous; tabouli.

Meat, Fish, Poultry, Legumes, Seeds, Nuts, and Meat Alternatives

Allowed: Fresh, plain meats, fish and poultry (no additives); whole fresh eggs; plain egg white substitute; dried beans such as chickpeas, split peas, kidney, navy, white, soy, and lentils; most nuts and seeds; plain tofu; peanut butter; gluten-free refried beans; homemade pizza made with allowed ingredients; soy milk that is malt-free or labeled gluten-free;

To Question: Processed or preserved meats such as luncheon meat, ham, bacon, canned meat, hot dogs, and sausage; prepared meatloaf or meatballs (unless you know ingredients); frozen or fresh meat patties; pate; imitation meats or fish products; meat product extenders; flavored egg white substitutes, dried eggs; canned baked beans; dry roasted nuts, flavored beer nuts; textured vegetable protein (TVP); frozen dinners; veggie or tofu burgers; other soy-based and/or tofu based foods; tempeh.

To Avoid: Fish or meat canned in vegetable broth containing hydrolyzed vegetable protein (HVP) or hydrolyzed plant protein (HPP) from ingredients not allowed; turkey basted or injected with HVP/HPP (if the plant source in HVP/HPP is not identified, or if the source is from wheat protein, HVP/HPP must be avoided); meat or fish prepared or thickened with unsafe flour, batter, or breadcrumbs; commercial pizza; seitan.

Soups

Allowed: Homemade soups and broth made with allowed ingredients.

To Question: Commercial canned or frozen prepared soups; dried soup mixes; canned broth; bouillon cubes; miso.

To Avoid: Soups made with ingredients not allowed such as barley, wheat pasta, and non-GF broths; soups thickened with wheat flour or other gluten-containing grains.

Fruits and Vegetables

Allowed: Fresh, frozen, and canned fruits; fresh, frozen, dried, and canned vegetables; vegetable and fruit juices.

To Question: Dried fruits; commercial fruit pie-filling; french fries (especially those in restaurants because of cross-contamination); vegetables in sauce; boxed potato products.

To Avoid: Vegetables in cream or sauce made with unsafe ingredients; fruit pies with wheat based pastry; scalloped or other creamy potatoes containing wheat flour; batter-dipped and breaded vegetables.

Fats

Allowed: Butter; margarine; vegetable oils (including canola); lard; shortening; homemade salad dressing made with allowed ingredients; mayonnaise.

To Question: Commercial salad dressing.

To Avoid: Packaged suet; gravy and cream sauces thickened with unsafe flours.

Condiments and Others

Allowed: Plain pickles, relish; olives; ketchup; plain mustard; pure herbs and spices; pure black pepper; all vinegars (except malt); salsa; pure horseradish; Tabasco sauce; sauces and gravies made with ingredients allowed; pure cocoa; pure baking chocolate; carob chips; chocolate chips; coconut; psyllium.

To Question: Worcestershire sauce; specialty mustards; barbecue sauce; soy sauce; teriyaki sauce; taco sauce; horseradish sauce; baking powder; tamari sauce; sauce mixes and other commercial sauces.

To Avoid: Mustard pickles (made from wheat flour); malt vinegar; sauces and gravies made from ingredients not allowed; communion wafers made with gluten.

Desserts and Sweets

Allowed: Homemade puddings, egg custard, gelatin desserts; cakes, cookies, pies, and pastries made with allowed ingredients; honey; jam; jelly; marmalade; corn syrup; maple syrup; molasses; brown or white sugar; sherbet; marshmallows; confectioner's or powdered sugar; GF licorice; chewing gum.

To Question: Ice cream; ice cream cones and waffle cones; Pudding or custard mixes; candies, chocolate bars (which are not pure and oftentimes contain other ingredients), commercial cake frosting.

To Avoid: Candies made with ingredients not allowed; any pastry such as cake, cookies, pies, etc. made with ingredients not allowed.

Beverages

Allowed: Tea; regular, decaffeinated, instant, or ground coffee; pure cocoa; soft drinks (both regular and diet); juice; cider; wines and sparkling wines; GF beer; champagne; cognac; grappa; sake; brandy; sherry; distilled alcoholic bev erages such as bourbon, light rum (double check dark and spiced rums); gin; scotch whisky; tequila; vermouth; and vodka; and pure liqueurs. (Distilled liquors, no matter from what grain they are made, contain no gluten due to the distillation process).

To Question: Instant tea; coffee substitutes; flavored cof fee; fruit-flavored drinks; chocolate drinks; chocolate mixes or flavorings; flavored and herbal teas; powdered ice tea; some soy and rice drinks; wine coolers and carbonated alcoholic beverages.

To Avoid: Beer, ale, stout, and lager; cereal and malted beverages; barley based cordial.

Snacks

Allowed: Plain popcorn; plain nuts and seeds; GF pretzels; GF chips.

To Question: Plain and flavored potato chips; corn chips; dry roasted nuts; plain and flavored tortilla chips; other flavored snack chips; pretzels; soy nuts; rice cakes.

To Avoid: Some flavored snack chips may contain gluten.

Keep in mind that the food lists in this chapter are *not* an all-inclusive. You should still read all food labels carefully and learn how to spot ingredients and additives with gluten. If you are not sure of an ingredient, do some research on it before eating the food product. Get to know the origin and the composition of certain ingredients. For example, some barbecue sauces or marinades may contain vinegar, so make sure it is the type of vinegar allowed on a gluten-free diet. Taking time to keep a written record of every-thing you learn will provide you with quick access to a reliable reference source. It will take some time but it will get easier to follow your gluten-free diet.

Once you are able to accept your new lifestyle, you will be able to move on and work on learning all you can. Do plenty of research, ask plenty of questions, and learn the many variables that may affect the ingredients in the food that you eat.

Q: Are there any non-food items that contain gluten?

There are non-food products that may contain gluten ingredients and can be sources of contamination. Some of these products include mouthwash; vitamin and mineral supplements; cosmetics; medications (both prescription and over-the-counter); toothpaste; stamps, envelopes, and other gummed labels. The single word "starch" on medications can mean any type of starch. As with any food products, be sure these products are gluten-free before using them.

Chapter 3

Children and Celiac Disease

Symptoms in Children

Celiac disease can occur any time from infancy well into adulthood. Children with celiac disease can have different types of symptoms than adults with the same disease. Babies with celiac disease thrive until gluten is introduced into the diet. At that point, symptoms begin to appear. Experts recommend that solid foods, including gluten-containing food, *not* be introduced into an infant's diet until he or she is 4 to 6 months of age. Research suggests that introducing gluten-containing foods earlier then 4 months old or later then 6 months old may predispose infants to celiac disease, with earlier exposure being more detrimental than later exposure. Research continues to support breastfeeding throughout the first year as a protective measure. The physical appearance of a child with celiac disease could include a bloated abdomen, pencil-thin arms and legs, and a flat buttocks due to malnourishment. Children might not always have obvious symptoms, as adults do. They tend to have poor appetites and become listless and irritable. Children with celiac disease frequently grow below their normal potential and some will actually stop growing completely. For some, this is the only symptom of the disease. X-rays of the bones usually show a lack of calcium and an overall slowing of bone growth. Children may become anemic (lack of iron in the blood) and pale. Vomiting and frequent diarrhea can also be typical symptoms. Children may also show damage to the enamel of their teeth. Teenagers may hit puberty at a later age and be shorter in stature. Celiac disease could cause some hair loss. The gluten-sensitive skin rash, dermatitis herpetiformis, is very uncommon in children.

Marcy Thorner from New Market, MD, shares the story of her daughter who is now in her early teens. Her daughter was a vigorous, active baby who changed suddenly into a lethargic, weight-losing, pale, and bloated infant. She refused to walk. She had once been running all over their 2-acre yard, jumping in leaf piles, in October 1993. By the spring of 1994, she wouldn't even walk across the driveway. Marcy spent five months carting her daughter around the house in her little red wagon, schlepping back and forth to the pediatrician for more tests and more head scratching. Finally, the doctor threw up his hands and sent them to a specialist at the National Children's Hospital in Washington, D.C. The doctor was quite dismissive of her daughter's symptoms until she needed a diaper change in his office, and, though he took one look at it and said "celiac disease," it still took another two months to get the final diagnosis. That was five months from the time she first detected symptoms and one month before her daughter turned 2 years old.

Diagnosis of the Child

Just as with adults, if children exhibit any of the symptoms of celiac disease, they should *not* be put on a gluten-free diet before testing has been done to properly diagnose their condition. A change in the child's diet will make the diagnosis more difficult. A diagnosis in children is similar to that of an adult and includes blood tests and a biopsy of the small intestines. As with adults, once the child is diagnosed with celiac disease, it is for life.

Treatment of the Child

After a child is properly diagnosed with celiac disease, the parent or caregiver must ensure that all food eaten by the child is gluten-free. The amount of fat and refined sugar that the child consumes should be limited for the first month after diagnosis because the lining of the intestines must be able to heal before these can be fully absorbed.

Total withdrawal of gluten from the child's diet will result in the disappearance of symptoms of the disease. For most, in a matter of days irritability diminishes and appetite improves. Within a few weeks, the child should begin to gain weight and diarrhea should decrease. Within several months, as the intestines heal and nutrients are again being absorbed, the child's growth should return to normal rates, abdominal bloating should disappear, and blood values should return to normal. Many of the improvements in health and physical appearance will even occur long before the intestinal damage has actually healed.

Challenges of a Child's Gluten-Free Diet

Children on a gluten-free diet will need extra special care and understanding. A child's body is geared toward eating to grow and develop properly. Feeding your child a diet that is both healthy and gluten-free is essential. Don't get in the habit of restricting yourself to cooking only a few easy recipes. Use as wide a range of gluten-free ingredients as possible. It is important that a child on a gluten-free diet not be made to feel different from other children. It will help if the whole family eats gluten-free meals. Choose recipes (such as those in Chapter 6) that are gluten-free and that the whole family can enjoy.

It is important that children always have plenty of support. As children enter the adolescent years, they may rebel and begin to refuse the diet. In these older children, if they begin to eat gluten-containing foods, symptoms may not appear right away although damage is being done to the intestines. This may deceive the child into thinking that he or she no longer needs a gluten-free diet and is cured when this is not really the case. Constant support and making sure the child's diet is never considered a nuisance is invaluable to how the child accepts his or her condition. Explain to your child, depending on his or her age and level of understanding, what the condition is and why it requires him or her to eat special foods. You would be surprised what children can understand at even the youngest ages. Explain it to them but don't make it an "issue." Explain it in a positive light and let them know they will be okay.

Preschool Children

One of the biggest challenges a parent faces is when friends or relatives tempt children with inappropriate foods. At a young age, children may not yet understand that they should not eat the food. You can watch them when they are at home, but they are exposed to food outside the home when they attend daycare, go to nursery school, visit babysitters, and visit family. It is difficult for the parent or caregiver to know if the child has consumed gluten, because it is the child that is going to experience the symptoms, and he or she may not tell you.

To make sure people know not to tempt your child when you are not around follow these tips:

- Pin a badge to your child that states, "I have a serious food allergy. Please do not feed me." Make it a fun colorful badge so people will notice it and the child won't mind wearing it. Even though your child does not have an actual food allergy it will get people's attention.

- Send a letter to anywhere your child may visit on a regular basis stating that your child has celiac disease and a list the foods he or she must avoid. Stress that not even a little bit is tolerable. Don't forget to include non-food items, such as play dough or glue, that your child may come in contact with.

- Teach caregivers how to read a basic food label ingredient list in order to decide if a snack or food is acceptable for your child to eat. Provide an extensive list all caregivers can use as a resource. Also explain contamination issues.

- Explain to the caregiver what type of symptoms your child may experience due to the condition and what action you would like taken in case symptoms arise.

- Reinforce the fact that your child is not sick but that he or she has a condition that requires a special diet. Stress that they try not to treat your child any different than the others in that respect.

Marcy Thorner worked out a special code with her daughter, Alix, when she was at this young age. She coined a phrase in the house called, "Special Alix Food," which she abbreviated "SAF." She used this abbreviation when she labeled food packages for the freezer or pantry. She bought butterfly stickers to put on the SAF items so that her daughter could select foods herself from the snack cupboard. By age 5, Marcy had her daughter starting to read ingredient labels in the grocery store. Now her daughter orders for herself in restaurants, asking the right questions and giving all the instructions about frying a burger in a clean pan instead of on the grill, no bun, and don't put anything else on the plate. Empowering your child by providing them the knowledge they need on gluten-free diets will give them the confidence they need to live a normal, healthy life.

Attending School

Children need to be taught along the way. As they get older, they need to be able to gradually begin to take control over their diet by knowing what to avoid, learning to read labels, and learning to make some of their own meals. It may be easier at this age to send your child to school with a lunch packed from home rather than suffering the difficulties of the cafeteria. If you have good support from the staff at school, you may want to let him or her purchase lunch in the cafeteria occasionally to help him or her feel like part of the crowd. When packing lunches, try sending ones that are similar to what the other children may be eating.

During this time it is still important to both send a letter and speak to the teacher, principal, school nurse, and school dietitian about your child's situation. Make sure to send a letter each year for new teachers or new school staff. The following is a sample letter that may help you to get started:

Dear Mr./Mrs./Ms. _____,

We are delighted to have Sally in your classroom and school this year.

Sally has a serious medical condition called celiac disease and must follow a medically prescribed diet. Over the past several years, we have found that good communication between the teacher, Sally, and ourselves is essential in managing her condition. Sally's condition requires a diet that is free of all gluten. If we can speak ahead of time about food-related work, birthdays, holiday celebrations, and field trips that involve food, I can either suggest a particular brand or substitution that may work for all the kids or I will send something for Sally to enjoy while the rest of the class eats what they have prepared. Please don't hesitate to call me at any time to let me know what you are planning, to check to see if something is okay for her, and to let me know how I can help.

In past years, we brought a snack tub for everyday treats that worked well. Sally made her own selections from the tub, and we replenished often. If that works well for you, I will bring one again this year. I am happy to do whatever I can to make things easier for you and to help Sally feel more in- cluded. Last year we pulled together a list of parent sign-ups for holiday parties and a class birthday list. On those days, I gave Sally the choice of bringing a special treat or eating from her snack tub. She seemed to do well having more control over how she wanted to manage the social situation. If that is pos- sible again this year, it helps Sally to take some responsibility for managing her own diet.

Attached is a list of products, by brand name, that she can have. All fresh fruits and vegetables, peanuts in the shell, and white milk are safe. The safety of processed foods and juices is complicated. Safe foods can become "contaminated" if they come into contact with gluten-containing foods, such as crumbs on a table or knife that was used to spread something on crackers.

If Sally is exposed to gluten, she will have stomach pain within 12 to 24 hours and very loose stools. She will need to use the bathroom urgently if she has eaten something she shouldn't have. We will certainly pick her up from school if you notice her holding her stomach or mentioning that it hurts. The pain only lasts for the day; however, the stools will con- tinue to be loose for up to a week. We appreciate knowing immediately if she has accidentally been exposed to gluten so we can watch for symptoms. Celiac disease is similar to an allergy in that she must avoid all foods and contact with ma- terials that contain gluten, which includes wheat, rye, barley, and their derivatives. Without contact with these products, Sally is fine and can participate in all activities. However, even a trace of gluten will cause serious damage. Sally can also react from skin contact with gluten. Although these things may not be part of your regular program, play dough, papier-mâché, stringing cereal or pasta, some glues and paints, or licking stickers or envelopes will expose her to gluten through skin contact.

I am happy to provide gluten-free substitutes for all of these materials or will call the manufacturer to verify gluten-free status of the products you now use.

We will send lunches for Sally on a daily basis. If you can provide us with a monthly lunch menu, it will help us to pattern what we send depending on what the other kids may be eating. Sometimes the lunches will be very similar to what the other kids are having, often they will be adapted slightly (different taco shell or hamburger without the bun), and occasionally Sally will have something entirely different.

Please call me at anytime if you have questions or concerns. Sally is aware of her condition and has adjusted well. She does well in an atmosphere of relaxed, knowledgeable, alert awareness of potentially unsafe conditions whenever food is available. I appreciate you providing the extra communication her special dietary needs require. It takes more time and I am very grateful for your efforts in keeping Sally both healthy and feeling included in class activities.

Sincerely,

Mr. and Mrs. XXX

(include phone number)

*Thank you to Lindsay Amadeo from Des Moines, IA, for her sample letter that contributed to this sample letter.

The Teenage Years

The teen years come with extra peer pressure to eat foods such as pizza or fast food burgers that need to be avoided. It is important to have taught your child how to hangout with friends without giving into peer pressure when it comes to eating. As long as they know the foods they can substitute so they can still hang out with friends at parties, restaurants, and dances, they will have the courage to stick with what they know is right.

Helpful Hints for Children of All Ages

These tips will help make social and educational events safe and fun for children with celiac diease:

- Make sure there is a gluten-free cake or other goodies at every birthday party. Drop it off before the other kids arrive and talk to the host.

- Consider sending your child to a gluten-free camp in the summertime. It can help your child meet other children who have celiac disease and help him or her feel less isolated. Check local support groups for camps in your area.

- Be sure all caregivers, teachers, principals, coaches, cafeteria personnel, friends, and friends' parents understand the necessity of your child sticking to a strict gluten-free diet.

- Both speak to and send letters to your child's teachers at the start of every school year. Be sure each teacher realizes that he or she must provide the information to any substitute teachers throughout the school year.

- Stress to any caregiver or teacher that the problem can go beyond meal issues. Discuss the problems of craft, art, or cooking projects for safety.

- Join a support group of other parents who have children on gluten-free diets.

- Keep plenty of gluten-free snacks in the house for children to grab at any time. This will help deter them from reaching for foods that contain gluten. Keep the gluten-free foods in accessible places and plainly labeled.

- Use brightly colored stickers to label gluten-free foods, making it easy for your child to identify and easy for anyone in the house who takes care of the child to identify.

- Have gluten-free foods available when you travel or go on family vacations.

- Involve your child in cooking and planning gluten-free meals.

- Involve your child in shopping for gluten-free foods and help him or her to learn how to read labels and quickly spot ingredients to avoid.

- Encourage your child to talk about his or her feelings concerning living with celiac disease.

- Begin teaching your child at an early age about how to manage his or her diet. Teach at whatever level you feel your child can understand. Incorporate the help of a dietitian that specializes in celiac disease.

- Empower your child by encouraging healthy caution instead of debilitating fear.

- Having the child wear a medical-alert bracelet or necklace can be a good reminder to anyone who may take care of your child in your absence.

- Maintain a supply of gluten-free, healthy snacks at your child's school, with the caregiver, grandparents or other family members, best friends, and anyone with whom the child may spend a good amount of time. The more safe and healthy snacks and foods you can provide your child with in places outside the home, the more accepting others will be and the more integrated your child's involvement with others will be.

- Be as involved as possible in your child's activities so that you are more able to monitor his or her food intake and sense of belonging. Do this by chaperoning trips and activites or being a den mother, scout leader, or teacher's assistant.

- Support your child in every way. He or she shouldn't feel reluctant to let you know about a reaction to a food out of fear of being disciplined or scolded. If the child does eat something that is harmful, instead of scolding, be supportive and helpful until the reaction subsides. Then, at the appropriate time, calmly discuss what happened and whether or not it was an accident. Explain the health consequences of these accidents.

- When your child is old enough, role-play situations that may come up in everyday life so that he or she will know how to handle such things as school, being at friends' houses, attending parties, or going out to eat. Share ideas for what to say to people when faced with various situations.

Marcy Thorner believes her daughter has a good foundation and overall an exceptional attitude. She states, "I have not let any doors close because of her condition. We cook together for fun. We travel. We eat out. She has attended Celiac Camp in Rhode Island. My goal is to help her become so self-confident and well-centered that she makes good decisions regardless of the pressure to conform that plagues teens. Through the years, I've developed a repertoire of simple family meals that require little or no adaptation to accommodate a strict gluten-free diet. I have a long list of tips and tricks that have made life easier, less expensive, less embarrassing for my child, and altogether more satisfying."

Meal Ideas for Children

These are only a few ideas for meals and snacks. Use your imagination and your children's likes and dislikes for adaptations. Their diets should include variety and foods that they enjoy.

Main Meals and Side Dishes

- GF hot dogs on homemade buns or rolled in a corn tortilla with GF cheese.
- GF pasta with GF tomato sauce
- Grilled GF cheese sandwich on GF bread
- GF bologna and GF cheese
- Homemade fish sticks
- GF cheese quesadilla on corn tortilla
- GF deli meat rolled in corn tortilla
- Homemade chicken nuggets
- Mini pizzas made on GF English muffins or GF bagels
- Peanut butter and jelly on GF bread or corn tortilla
- GF beef or chicken tacos
- Homemade chili with GF corn chips
- GF waffles with peanut butter and jelly
- Corn-on-the cob
- GF baked beans
- Homemade hamburger on GF bun with GF cheese
- Homemade GF macaroni and cheese
- Homemade French fries

Snacks

- Cottage cheese and fruit
- Applesauce

- Cold GF cereal
- GF fruited yogurt or plain, unflavored yogurt topped with fruit
- GF string cheese
- GF rice cakes with peanut butter
- Fresh fruit, cut-up or whole
- Canned fruit such as fruit cocktail, pineapple chunks, or peaches
- Microwave popcorn
- Homemade pudding
- Hard-boiled egg
- Fresh veggies such as carrot sticks or baby carrots, celery sticks, or cherry tomatoes
- Celery with peanut butter
- Apple with peanut butter
- GF Chips (many flavors of GF chips are available at the grocery store)
- Raisins
- GF corn nuts
- Milkshake made with GF ingredients
- Jell-O, plain or with fruit
- GF pretzels
- Marshmallows
- GF cookies
- Fruit smoothies

Resources for Children

There are many different resources and support groups set up for children who have celiac disease and their families. One of the most well-known support groups is R.O.C.K. (Raising Our Celiac Kids). Raising Our Celiac Kids is a support group for parents, families, and friends of kids with celiac disease or gluten intolerance. This group also welcomes families of autistic kids involved in a gluten-free/casein-free dietary intervention program. As their Website states, they concentrate on dealing with unique challenges that include:

- Finding fun gluten-free treats for kids.
- Menu ideas for school lunches, quick dinners, and sports snacks.
- Helping kids to take responsibility for reading labels, cooking, and planning and preparing food.
- How to prepare for unexpected birthday parties and food-oriented activities at school, church, and elsewhere.
- Halloween, Easter, and other special days.
- Educating daycare providers and teachers without burdening them.
- Dealing with grandparents, babysitters, and "helpful" friends who offer gluten-containing foods to kids.
- Ensuring kids won't cheat, and what to do when they do.
- Sending kids away to camp, friends' houses, and other times when we're not around to help.
- The psychological impact of growing up with celiac disease (peer pressure, teenage years, etc.).

Danna Korn founded the group R.O.C.K. in 1991 after her son was diagnosed with celiac disease. The group has grown to international proportions and helps families all over the world deal with the unique challenges of raising a child on a gluten-free diet.

R.O.C.K. helps give these families the support they need in dealing with the feelings associated with the diagnosis and dealing with all aspects of the diet itself. It always helps to have some type of guidance when initially tackling the gluten-free diet. People are invited to contact R.O.C.K. via e-mail at rock@celiackids.com or *www.celiackids.com.*

Chapter 4

The Gluten-Free Kitchen

Stocking Your Kitchen

It is a great idea to clear out a special cupboard in the kitchen to store all the special products you will need for the gluten-free diet. Making sure you always have certain products on hand will make whipping up meals and snacks much easier. You can make things even easier by batch cooking. Cook large quantities of food or dishes and freeze the leftovers in individual storage containers to allow for a quick and easy meal or snack.

People on gluten-free diets often need to cook from scratch to ensure that meals and dishes are, in fact, gluten-free. Cooking from scratch does not have to be so time-consuming. There are several kitchen appliances you can use to help reduce your workload. Bread-makers, heavy-duty mixers, Crock-Pots, and pasta makers can be very helpful additions to the gluten-free kitchen.

As with any type of diet, it is wise to plan ahead when on a gluten-free diet. Having the following foods on hand will ensure no-hassle preparation when it is time for a meal or snack.

Gluten-Free Kitchen Essentials
- Assorted jams and jellies
- Baking powder (GF, such as Clabber Girl or Calumet)

- Baking soda
- Beans: chickpeas, kidney beans, lentils, GF refried beans, GF baked beans
- Breads: GF bread, bagels, buns, waffles, and/or muffins
- Bread crumbs (GF)
- Bread machine
- Bouillon base and cubes (GF)
- Canned chicken (GF)
- Canned tuna or salmon (GF)
- Cereal (GF)
- Cheese (GF)
- Condiments (relish, GF ketchup, etc.)
- Cookbooks
- Cornstarch, potato starch, tapioca starch
- Corn tortillas or tacos
- Cottage cheese
- Crackers (GF)
- Cream of tartar
- Crock pot
- Eggs (whole, fresh)
- Flours such as bean flour, chickpea flour, millet flour, potato starch flour, brown/white rice flour, sorghum flour, soy flour, sweet rice flour, and/or tapioca flour
- Fresh and/or frozen fruit
- Fresh meats
- Fresh and/or frozen vegetables
- Fruit juices
- Herbs and pure spices (such as garlic powder, onion powder, pure black pepper)
- Honey

- Margarine or butter
- Milk (low fat or fat free)
- Mixes for GF bread, muffins, waffles, cakes, and brownies
- Nuts and seeds
- Onions
- Pasta (GF such as rice, corn, potato, legume, quinoa)
- Peanut butter
- Popcorn, plain or GF microwave popcorn
- Potatoes (whole)
- Pretzels (GF such as Glutino Brand)
- Rice (brown)
- Rice cakes: GF mini flavored rice cakes or large version
- Salad dressings (GF)
- Sauces (GF): BBQ sauce, pizza sauce, pasta sauce, salsa, soy sauce, teriyaki sauce
- Seeds and nuts (almonds, peanuts, walnuts, sunflower seeds, sesame seeds)
- Sugar (white and brown)
- Tofu (plain)
- Tomato paste, whole tomatoes, diced tomatoes, tomato sauce (GF)
- Vanilla
- Vegetable oil
- Vinegar: white and red wine, cider, rice and balsamic
- Xanthan gum or guar gum
- Yogurt: plain or GF fruited yogurt

All About Gluten-Free Flours

There are plenty of gluten-free mixes on the market today that are perfect for breads, muffins, biscuits, cakes, and any of your favorite baked goods, but you can still bake from scratch if your heart so desires. It just takes a little extra work when baking with gluten-free flours. Many health food stores, specialty online gluten-free stores, and even local grocery stores sell gluten-free flours and/or flour mixtures. There are many types of flours that are gluten-free, but the typical ones include corn, rice, soy, tapioca, potato starch flour, or a mixture of these.

Using these types of flours in place of wheat flour may give foods a different taste and texture so practice and experiment with them to find the right combination. There are all types of cookbooks that can provide you with detailed information about gluten-free baking along with scrumptious recipes.

The following is a list of some of the types of gluten-free flours.

Amaranth: Mild nut-like flavor and good for baking, it is best when used in combination with other gluten-free flours.

Arrowroot flour: No real flavor, typically used as a thickener in many foods, similar in texture to corn starch and can be exchanged for cornstarch, measure for measure, in recipes and mixes.

Brown rice flour: Slightly sweet, mild flavor, and excellent for use in desserts, it has a higher nutrient content (including fiber) than white rice flour and contains bran. Use it in combination with other gluten-free flours as a type of binding agent (such as eggs, mashed banana, or applesauce) to avoid a crumbly end product. Best used for breads, muffins, and cookies where a bran or nutty flavor is desired. Due to the oils in the bran, this flour has a short shelf life and its flavor will become stronger as it ages. Pur chase it fresh and store it in the refrigerator or freezer to preserve it longer.

Buckwheat flour: Strong flavored, best when used in small quantities in combination with other gluten-free flours. Even though it has wheat in the name it is gluten-free and not related to wheat—it is instead related to the rhubarb plant. Be aware that some companies mix buckwheat flour with wheat flour to lessen its strong taste so always check.

Chickpea flour: Hearty but mild flavor, made from garbanzo beans, and high in protein and fiber, it can be used in combination with other gluten-free flours and when baking.

Corn flour: Milled from corn (maize), has a mild corn taste, and adds a light texture to baked goods, it is great for blending with cornmeal to make corn bread or corn muffins and best when used in combination with other gluten-free flours.

Garfava flour: A blend of garbanzo and fava beans, developed by Authentic Foods, it is high in protein and fiber, and it creates excellent volume and moisture content in baked goods.

Millet flour: Because it tends to make breads dry and course, substitute only 1/5 of the flour mixture with this flour.

Nut or legume flours: Nutty in flavor, it can be used in small portions to enhance the taste of puddings, cookies, or homemade pasta.

Potato flour: Not the same as potato starch flour and heavier in texture, it is best when used in small quantities and combined with other gluten-free flours, and should be stored in the refrigerator or freezer.

Potato starch flour: Made from potatoes, this fine white flour keeps well and is excellent for baking if sifted several times and used in recipes that include eggs. It can also be utilized as a thickener.

Rice polish: Soft, fluffy, and cream-colored, this flour is made from the hulls of brown rice. Much like rice bran and high in nutritive value, it has a short shelf life. Buy it fresh and store in the refrigerator or freezer.

Sorghum flour: A fairly new product ground from specialty bred sorghum grain, it is best used in combination with other gluten-free flours, stores well on the pantry shelf, and can be substituted for rice flour.

Soy flour: Smooth textured and nutty in flavor, its de fatted type is lower in fat and will store longer. Soy flour should be stored in the refrigerator or freezer (due to its shorter shelf life), is best when used in combination with other gluten-free flours because of its strong flavor, and has a high nutritive content. If you are sensitive to soy, bean flour can be substituted for soy flour in most recipes.

Sweet rice flour: Called "sticky rice" and made from a glutinous rice, this is an excellent thickening agent, especially in sauces that are to be refrigerated or frozen. Not the same as plain white rice flour, it helps to bind ingredients together when baking.

Tapioca starch flour: A light tasteless flour that comes from the root of the cassava plant, it adds a "chew" factor to baked goods, is excellent for thickening soups, creams, gravies, puddings, and gravies. It can be stored on the pantry shelf for long periods of time.

Teff flour: A versatile grain with a mild, nutty, and slightly sweet flavor, it can be a great thickener in soups, gravies, stews and pudding.

Quinoa flour: Slightly bitter in flavor, this makes excellent biscuits and pancakes.

White rice flour: Not much flavor or nutrition, it has a long shelf life, and is best used in combination with other gluten-free flours.

Whole bean flour or Romano bean flour: Dark and strong in taste, these flours are milled from the Romano or cranberry bean. They are high in fiber, protein, and other nutrients. Products made with these flours are denser and require less for best results.

Other Flour Combinations

Both of these flour mixtures have a long shelf life and can be stored at room temperature. A cup of this flour mix is equal to one cup of wheat flour. This blend is also known as Bette Hagman's "Gluten-Free Gourmet Original Blend" and is very popular. It is a heavy mix but will exchange well, cup for cup, with wheat flour when you are adapting recipes. Because of its low protein content, the mix calls for adding extra protein and/or leavening, such as egg whites, dry milk powder, gelatin, or an egg replacer.

Bette Hagman´s Gluten-Free Gourmet Original Blend

Makes 3 cups

2 cups white rice flour

1/3 cup tapioca/starch flour

2/3 cup potato starch flour

This flour is available already mixed through Ener-g Foods at *www.ener-g.com*.

Another great blend called, Bette Hagman's "Four Flour Blend" also exchanges cup for cup with wheat flour. This mix does have enough protein so you should not have to add extra. The only other addition you would have to make when adapting your recipe is xanthan gum.

Bette Hagman´s Four Flour Blend

Makes 3 cups

2/3 cup Garfava bean flour

1 cup cornstarch

1/3 cup sorghum flour

1 cup tapioca/starch flour

This flour is also available already mixed through Authentic Foods and can be purchased at *www.glutenfree-supermarket.com*.

One more wonderful flour mix is Bette Hagman's "Featherlight Blend," which also exchanges cup for cup with wheat flour. This particular blend contains enough protein and fiber to use in regular cookies and cake recipies without changing anything but the addition of xanthan gum. This makes a great blend for baking gluten-free breads and buns.

Bette Hagman's Featherlight Blend

Makes 3 cups

1 cup rice flour

1 cup cornstarch

1 cup tapioca/starch flour

1 Tbsp. potato flour

This flour is also available already mixed through Authentic Foods and can be purchased at *www.glutenfree-supermarket.com*.

The Bette Hagman flour recipes are from *The Gluten-Free Gourmet Living Well Without Wheat, Revised Edition* by Bette Hagman (Henry Holt and Company, LLC, 2000).

Substitutions for Wheat Flour as a Thickener*

Gluten-free flours, starches, and other ingredients can be used as thickening agents in sauces, soups, stews, gravy, puddings, and other food items. Each has its own unique properties, therefore some are more suitable than others for thickening. Starches should be mixed in cold water before using, added during the last five minutes of cooked and not overcooked. Flours should also be mixed in cold liquid before using. Gelatin needs to be softened in cold water, heated until the liquid is clear and then added to the food item to be thickened. Cooked starches are more clear and shiny, whereas cooked flours are more cloudy and opaque in appearance.

Substitution for 1 Tbsp. Wheat Flour

Starches	
Amaranth Starch	1 1/2 tsp.
Arrowroot Starch	1 1/2 tsp.
Cornstarch	1 1/2 tsp.

Substitution for 1 Tbsp. Wheat Flour, Continued	
Flours	
Bean (garbanzo/chickpea)	1 Tbsp.
Brown Rice Flour	1 Tbsp.
Sweet Rice Flour	1 Tbsp.
Tapioca Flour	1 Tbsp.
White Rice Flour	1 Tbsp.
Others	
Gelatin Powder	1 1/2 tsp.
Quick-Cooking Tapioca	2 tsp.

*Used with permission from: *Gluten-Free Diet: A Comprehensive Resource Guide* (October 2008), by Shelley Case, RD, Case Nutrition Consulting, Inc., *www.glutenfreediet.ca*.

It is important to add either guar gum or xanthan gum to your gluten-free baked goods to compensate for the lack of gluten. This will add texture and affect the appearance of the overall food. When using xanthan or guar gum, the basic formula for breads or pizza is 1 to 2 teaspoon per cup of flour; for cakes 1/2 to 1 teaspoon per cup of flour, and for most cookies 1/4 to 1/2 teaspoon per cup of flour. Each recipe will call for different amounts but this is a good rule of thumb to use if you are not sure.

Food Item	Suitable Thickeners
Cream Soups	Amaranth starch, bean flour, rice flour (brown, sweet, white), tapioca flour
Fruit Sauces	Arrowroot starch, cornstarch, sweet rice flour
Fruit Pies and Cobblers	Cornstarch, quick-cooking tapioca
Gravy	Rice flour (brown, sweet, white), tapioca flour
Puddings	Amaranth starch, cornstarch, gelatin, sweet rice flour
Savory Sauces	Amaranth starch, arrowroot starch, bean flour, cornstarch, sweet rice flour
Stews	Bean flour, rice flour, (brown, sweet, white), tapioca flour
Stir-Fry Dishes	Arrowroot starch, cornstsarch, tapioca flour

*Used with permission from: *Gluten-Free Diet: A Comprehensive Resource Guide* (October 2008), by Shelley Case, RD, Case Nutrition Consulting, Inc., *www.glutenfreediet.ca.*

Keep in mind that some gluten-free flours are very perishable. Store them in an airtight container in the freezer or refrigerator and label them with the date you made them so you can keep track of how long you have stored them.

When you are in need of a gluten-free baking powder try the following:

 ## Gluten-Free Baking Powder

1/3 cup baking soda

2/3 cup arrowroot or potato starch

2/3 cup cream of tartar

Mix well and store in an airtight container.

1 1/2 tsp. of this mixture is equal to 1 tsp. of regular baking powder.

Tips for the Gluten-Free Baker and Cook

The following tips are essential to remember when cooking and baking gluten-free foods. Some of the tips have been adapted from Shelly Case's *Gluten-Free Diet: A Comprehensive Resource Guide, Expanded and Revised Edition.*

- Start with simple recipes until you have mastered the art of cooking with gluten-free flours and products.

- Modify your favorite recipes by substituting gluten-free flours and other ingredients. Try starting with recipes that already incorporate gluten-free flours.

- Most gluten-free flours do not substitute cup for cup with wheat flour, so use the chart on pages 83 and 84 to substitute the correct amounts.

- When you substitute gluten-free flour for wheat flour, you will usually get the best results with recipes that call for only a small amount of flour (less than 2 cups).

- Recipes that call for cake flour will do well when substituted with gluten-free flour.

- Gluten-free flours require using more leavening agents in the recipe than with wheat flours. Add a little extra GF baking powder and/or baking soda to boost rising properties of your product.

- Baked goods turn out better when combinations of gluten-free flours are used. Brown or white rice flour plus potato starch flour and tapioca works well in breads. Potato starch flour plus cornstarch work well in pizza dough, and white rice flour plus tapioca works well for cakes.

- Put a pan of water in the oven when you are baking your product to help keep in the moisture.

- When using glass-baking dishes, reduce the oven temperature by 25 degrees.

- For extra flavor and moisture try adding nuts, fruits (such as applesauce, pureed pumpkin or mashed banana), dried fruits (such as raisins), GF yogurt, or honey. Also try adding a little extra oil or shortening if you feel your recipes are too dry.

- Adding nut meal (finely ground walnuts, pecans, almonds) in baked goods adds an amazing amount of moisture and a unique taste.

- Quinoa flakes can substitute for oatmeal in recipes if gluten-free rolled oats are not available or tolerated.

- Sift your flour and mixes before and after measuring them. This will help to improve texture.

- Add an extra egg or egg white for improved smoothness and crumb structure.

- Use Knox or any other unflavored gelatin in your baking recipes to help add moisture and help bind the ingredients. Before adding, mix the powder with half the water called for in the recipe.

- Beat gluten-free breads by hand with a wooden spoon or spatula. The batter or dough is usually too thick for a whisk. This keeps it from being over-beaten and from becoming too fine and falling when baked.

- Using smaller pans will yield a better product. Try using bun rings, muffin tins, bunt pans, and very small bread pans. If you can't find the right size or shape try using aluminum foil and folding it into the shape that you want.

- Use 1 1/2 tsp. cream of tartar and 1 tsp. baking soda for two loaves of bread. It will not interfere with the yeast and will help the bread to rise and help to keep it up during the baking process.

- When baking cookies, refrigerate the cookie sheet for half an hour before baking them to help keep the cookies from spreading too much.

- Refrigerate gluten-free dough for at least half an hour or, better yet, overnight to help soften the dough for a better textured product.

- Try replacing a small amount (about 1 Tbsp.) of gluten-free flour with glutinous rice or sweet rice flour for baked goods such as brownies.

- Try substituting buttermilk for milk or water in gluten-free breads. This can result in a lighter and more finely textured product.

- Cornstarch and tapioca work the best for thickening foods such as sauces and gravies.

- To bind meat loaf or meatballs, try using plain popcorn that is blended into crumbs.

Choosing a Bread Machine

Bread machines have become quite popular through the years, though not all machines are suited for making gluten-free breads. Some people prefer to use them whereas others prefer to make bread by hand. If you decide to invest in one, keep some of these important features in mind:

- Because gluten-free dough is heavier and harder to mix, choose a machine that has larger paddles.

- If the machine has an oblong, loaf-shaped pan, choose one that has two large paddles instead of one large paddle in the center. This will prevent the need to continually scrape the corners during the kneading process.

- Find a model that can be programmed for one rising cycle.

- Find a model that allows you to switch manually from knead to rise to bake, thus allowing you to manually control all the cycles.

- Gluten-free bread is usually made on the short or rapid cycle of the machine. Some of the machines will mix only once on this setting; others may mix twice. To get the best use out of your machine, you should be able to stop it at the dough stage and take the dough out so you can use it for other things besides bread.

- Find a model that has a cool-down cycle so the bread will not become soggy if it sits in the pan without being removed immediately.

- If you choose not to freeze bread, look for a model that offers a smaller bucket for a smaller size loaf.

There are many different types of bread machines on the market today. Talk to others who bake with them and ask for their recommendations.

Keep these tips in mind when baking bread with your bread machine:

- If there is dry flour sitting on the top of or in the corners of the dough, then it probably needs more liquid and/or better mixing. Add warm water (1 tsp. at a time), mixing after each addition, until the dough is smooth and less dry.

- If the dough is too thin (the consistency of cake batter) and has no defined lines on top, then it probably needs more dry ingredients. Add 1 Tbsp. of rice flour at a time, stirring after each incorporation, until the dough is thicker and will pull away from the sides.

- Use flour and eggs that are at room temperature.

- Use warm ingredients (not hot) to help the bread to rise.

- Use milk and butter, instead of water and oil, to add moisture to the bread and create a chewy crust.

Preventing Cross-Contamination

Not only is it important to make sure you check for gluten in the ingredients of the foods you eat, but it is also just as important to be aware of possible cross-contamination with gluten-containing foods. This happens when a gluten-free product somehow comes into contact with something that contains gluten. At home, contamination can occur when your foods are prepared on common surfaces or when utensil or appliances are not cleaned thoroughly after use with a gluten-containing food. On an even larger scale, contamination can occur in manufacturing plants if separate machines are not used or if thorough cleaning does not take place between the production of batches. It is important to minimize cross-contamination as much as possible. It doesn't take much for the intestinal villi of the person with celiac disease to become damaged with small amounts of gluten-containing foods. There are several simple steps that can help reduce the chances for cross-contamination, some adapted from *Gluten-Free Diet: A Comprehensive Resource Guide- Expanded and Revised Edition.*

Implement a "no double-dipping" rule in your household. An example of "double-dipping" is when a knife is dipped into a spreadable type condiment (such as peanut butter, jelly, mayonnaise, margarine), spread on the bread, and then dipped into the condiment again. The condiment becomes contaminated with the gluten-containing crumbs. Squeeze bottles can make a safe alternative. You can also make it a rule to have the family use a spoon to get condiments out of the container and then spread it with a knife, stressing that they be careful not to touch the spoon to the bread. If other family members can't seem to stop double-dipping, buy separate condiments and label them as gluten-free and non-gluten-free. You can buy one large container of a product and then divide it into two smaller containers to save money. Label each container so you know which is gluten-free. If the family uses up the non-gluten-free jar first and there is still quite a bit left in the gluten-free jar, give it to them to use up more quickly. When making any type of dip, put some aside for the person who is eating gluten-free if non-gluten-free food will be dipped into the main batch.

Pay special attention to the instruments and containers used to prepare and store food. Designate certain appliances for use only with gluten-free products. Toasters can be a popular source of contamination because of the crumbs it can collect. Either designate a slot in the toaster that is only for gluten-free bread or buy a separate toaster for gluten-free products. Using a toaster oven that has a shelf that can be wiped clean after each use can also work. Be sure to wash utensils, cutting boards, other surfaces, pots, and pans thoroughly after each use. Also, wipe counters right before use, because wheat flours can stay airborne for many hours and contaminate exposed preparation surfaces and utensils.

Store gluten-free products in separate labeled containers. You may even want to place gluten-free products in a separate cupboard and designated shelf in the refrigerator. You can use colored labels or other types of labels to help make sure everyone in the family as well as caregivers know which products are gluten-free. Do not share nonstick and cast iron cookware with gluten-containing foods. They can be very porous. A better choice is stainless steel cookware. Use aluminum foil on baking sheets or pans that are also used for foods containing gluten. Purchase a separate colander for your gluten-free pastas. This is safer because it is quite hard to get colanders completely cleaned, even in the dishwasher.

When preparing gluten-free and non-gluten-free foods at the same time (such as pasta), make sure you use separate utensils and food preparation tools. It may be easier to prepare one at a time. In fact it may be better to purchase a separate set of utensils and other items needed for gluten-free cooking and baking. This might include buying separate paddles and bowls if you have a bread machine that is used for both regular and gluten-free breads. Tell caregivers who may be in the house how and why separate foods are needed. Stress the importance of not mixing foods, utensils, and/or appliances. Avoid buying products such as flour from bulk bins. Scoops that have been used in bins with gluten-containing products could contaminate the gluten-free products.

Care must be taken when eating at restaurants. Be aware that french fries (even though they might be gluten-free) may have been fried in the same oil that battered gluten-containing foods have been fried in, which will cause contamination. Specifically ask if the cook can clean the grill before preparing your foods and to keep your meal away from other meals that might contain gluten. You may want to call ahead to the restaurant to make sure it can handle your request. Be extra careful at buffet or family style restaurants because utensils being used in more than one serving pan can contaminate serving spoons.

Chapter 5

Preparing Everyday Gluten-Free Meals

Planning Ahead

Meal planning for the gluten-free diet means one thing: planning ahead. There are many foods that are naturally gluten-free, which means there are many foods you don't have to give up. There are even more of your favorite foods (such as pasta, bread, and baked goods) that can be made from gluten-free grains and taste pretty close to the foods you are used to. If you have a stocked kitchen and the foods that you need, you can make tasty, easy meals and snacks at any time.

Start with safe food choices, such as fresh meats, fresh fruits and vegetables, eggs, cheese, rice, potato products, and corn. Avoid flours made from wheat, rye, barley, and any derivative of these flours. Avoid breads, rolls, croutons, bread crumbs, cakes, pies, cookies, muffins, noodles, crackers, and cracker crumbs made with gluten-containing flours. Avoid soups, sauces, gravies, and batters that may be thickened with these flours. To help you get started, use some of the menu ideas in this chapter, but remember only to use this as a *starting point* to developing your own favorite meals and snacks.

The following is an excerpt on meal planning, used with permission, from "The Newly-Diagnosed Celiac and DH'er: Step-By-Step: Beginning the Gluten-Free Lifestyle" (*www.houstonceliacs.org*) by Janet Y. Rinehart and Lynn Rainwater:

- Plan meals before you get to the grocery store. The first couple of months will be frustrating when going grocery shopping, because you are new at reading labels, and, yes, gluten-free specialty products are more expensive. It's just a fact.

- To save time and trouble, plan on making as much of the meal gluten-free as possible. The person with celiac disease will appreciate not feeling different, and the cook will not have to make two meals. The "civilians" in the family can add gluten-containing bread or dessert items as they want.

- Start with simple meals, rather than combination dishes.

- Pay attention to all food sensitivities of your family. Make a rough draft of your meals for the next week, taking into consideration the family's schedule. Plan for the main entree, vegetables, fruit, and salad. Plan one new, interesting gluten-free dessert each week.

- Use the Celiac Sprue Association's *Gluten-Free Product List* to evaluate brand names of products (*www.csaceliacs.org*). Then make a brand-name grocery list based on the recipes you plan to use. Working on a weekly basis helps you eliminate extra trips to the grocery store, which will, in turn, reduce the frustration of looking at labels again and may save money.

- Be sure to plan for the family's snacks, both gluten-free and non-gluten-free. When you have gluten-free items readily available (such as nuts, popcorn, fruit, and raw cut-up vegetables), you will be less tempted to "cheat" when you are starving.

- Try at least one new gluten-free recipe a week. Mark your cookbooks with comments, or develop a list of your favorites with the cookbook page noted. Include the family in meal-planning. What kind of meals do they like? Try to find good gluten-free substitutes.

- Make good use of your freezer. Freeze single portions of dinners to use as lunch items. Freeze dessert items for snacks.

- There are many companies that manufacture gluten-free specialty products. These products are more expensive than the comparable; that's just a fact. However, many of the mixes, frozen meals, and already-baked goods are quite good and make your life easier. See the CSA/USA Gluten-Free Product Listing for a listing of some of the specialty food manufacturers (*www.csaceliacs.org*).

- There are several online grocery stores with extensive gluten-free product lists. You may want to consult support group members to get their opinion of some of the products before you invest in a big order.

- ALWAYS READ LABELS!

The Essential Gluten-Free Grocery Guide, which can be found at *www.triumphdining.com*, and Cecilia's Marketplace Gluten-Free Grocery Shopping Guide (*www.ceciliasmarketplace.com*) are good tools to help you to develop shopping lists of gluten-free products.

Meal and Snack Ideas

Start Your Day Out Right: Breakfast Ideas

- GF cold cereal with fat-free milk; sliced fresh fruit; juice.
- GF crepes filled with fresh fruit.

- Pancakes made from a GF mix or homemade GF batter; sliced strawberries; syrup; fruit juice.
- Hard-boiled egg; home fried potatoes; GF toast; fat-free milk; fresh fruit.
- GF muffin and fresh fruit.
- GF hot cereal (such as cream of rice or cream of buckwheat) topped with raisins and cinnamon; fat-free milk; 1/2 of a grapefruit.
- Fruit smoothie made from GF yogurt, skim milk, and fresh fruit blended together.
- GF toasted bagel with peanut butter; GF yogurt mixed with blueberries; fruit juice.
- Breakfast sandwich made from GF English muffin, scrambled egg, GF cheese, and GF ham; fruit juice.
- Homemade hash browns cooked and mixed with scrambled eggs, GF cheese, onions, and bell peppers; fruit juice or fresh fruit salad.
- Scrambled eggs with GF cheese and GF turkey sausage.

Time for a Lunch Break: Lunch Ideas

- Corn tortilla wrapped around homemade tuna salad; fresh fruit salad.
- Tuna melt sandwich made with tuna, GF bread, and GF cheese.
- Homemade chili topped with GF sour cream; GF corn chips; tossed salad with GF salad dressing; grapes.
- Homemade egg salad on toasted GF bagel; fresh fruit; GF yogurt.
- Baked potato topped with GF cheese, broccoli, and GF salsa; tossed salad with GF dressing.
- GF English muffin topped with GF pizza sauce, GF mozzarella cheese, and any vegetable toppings

you choose, toasted in an oven; tossed salad with GF dressing.

- Hearty green salad made with your favorite raw vegetables, GF cheese, sunflower seeds, hard boiled egg, grilled chicken breast, and GF salad dressing; served with a GF bread stick brushed with margarine and garlic powder and heated in the oven.

- Corn tortilla filled with chopped grilled chicken, GF cheddar cheese, GF salsa, diced tomatoes, and GF sour cream.

- GF soup (canned or homemade); grilled cheese and tomato sandwich made with GF bread.

- Homemade chicken salad served on top of mixed greens; GF roll with margarine.

- Homemade hummus on GF crackers; fresh vegetables dipped in GF ranch dressing.

- GF hot dog cut up and mixed into GF baked beans; carrot sticks and GF ranch dressing.

- GF hot dog rolled in a corn tortilla with your favorite toppings.

- Hamburger topped with grilled onions and GF cheese, served on a GF bun; GF tortilla chips and GF salsa.

- Cottage cheese served with fresh, sliced peaches.

- Homemade GF pasta salad and fresh fruit.

Super Suppers: Dinner Ideas

- Rice pasta cooked in olive oil with onions, peppers, mushrooms, broccoli, and fresh tomatoes; plain tofu, seafood, or your favorite meat.

- Barbecue pork or chicken using GF sauce; risotto with toasted almonds and broccoli.

- Grilled chicken breast topped with GF sharp cheddar cheese and GF salsa; brown rice mixed with GF salsa and steamed broccoli.

- Enchiladas made with corn tortillas and chicken or plain tofu.

- Chicken quesadilla made with grilled chicken and GF cheese between two corn tortillas, lightly brown on both sides in large fry pan sprayed with GF cooking spray, topped with GF salsa, GF sour cream, lettuce, and diced tomatoes.

- GF pasta mixed with lean ground beef or ground turkey, cooked zucchini, and GF spaghetti sauce; tossed salad with GF salad dressing; GF garlic bread.

- Pizza on GF crust or corn tortilla topped with your favorite meats, vegetables, and GF cheeses; tossed salad and GF dressing.

- Grilled salmon, swordfish, or halibut drizzled with mixture of GF soy sauce, honey, ginger, and garlic powder; red potatoes; fresh asparagus.

- Shish kabobs made with your favorite meat and vegetables (such as steak, chicken, shrimp, bell peppers, onion, mushrooms, tomatoes, or zucchini) marinated in GF Italian dressing and GF Teriyaki sauce, and cooked on the grill.

- Lean cut of steak cooked on the grill; baked sweet potato topped with margarine; steamed vegetables; tossed salad with GF dressing.

- Ground beef cooked with GF taco seasoning and topped with GF shredded cheddar cheese, chopped lettuce and tomatoes, black beans, chopped avocados, GF salsa, and GF sour cream, served in corn tortillas, corn taco shells, or over corn tortilla chips.

- Homemade meatloaf; garlic and cheese mashed potatoes (homemade mashed potatoes mixed with GF cheddar cheese and garlic powder to taste); steamed green beans.

- Homemade chili; GF corn bread; tossed salad with GF dressing.
- Beef, chicken, shrimp, or plain tofu stir-fried with GF soy sauce, your favorite vegetables and bean sprouts, served over brown rice.
- Lasagna made with GF pasta and GF ingredients; tossed salad with GF dressing.
- Homemade hamburger grilled and topped with cooked onions and GF cheese on a GF bun; GF baked beans; fresh vegetables and GF ranch dressing.
- Chicken fried steak made with GF flour; steamed vegetables; potatoes and onions fried in olive oil.
- Homemade stuffed peppers; tossed salad with GF dressing.

Got the Munchies?: Snack Ideas

- GF corn chips
- GF string cheese
- Raisins or other dried fruit
- Popcorn
- Plain corn nuts
- Hard boiled egg or deviled eggs
- Celery with cream cheese or peanut butter
- Fresh vegetables and GF ranch salad dressing
- Fresh fruit
- GF bread with peanut butter
- Homemade chocolate pudding topped with bananas
- Fruited gelatin made with fresh or GF canned fruit
- GF crackers and GF cheese

- GF rice cakes
- Applesauce sprinkled with cinnamon
- Homemade trail mix made from peanuts, plain M&Ms, raisins, and chocolate
- GF chips
- Apple with peanut butter
- Nuts and/or seeds (plain)
- GF yogurt and fruit
- Fruit smoothie

Favorite Meals From the Experts

The following are meal ideas from people who have celiac disease who wanted to share some of their favorites. Thanks everyone!

From Regina Celano of Ronkonkoma, New York

Chili Potato

Microwave a baking potato. Top it with Hormel Chili with beans (or any GF chili) and GF shredded cheddar cheese. Microwave again until cheese is melted.

Tex Mex Salad

Place some bagged salad mix on a plate. Microwave GF chili and pour over the salad. Top with GF shredded cheddar cheese, GF salsa, and GF sour cream. Dip GF tortilla chips into the mixture.

Pizza

Take a frozen Chebe Bread Pizza Crust out of the freezer. (When you make them, make several and freeze some for future use). Top with GF pizza sauce, GF shredded cheese, and any other GF pizza topping of your choice. Pop in the oven and dinner is served!

Chicken Salad Platter

Serve a chicken salad made using GF ingredients over bagged salad. Serve with some cheesy Parmesan bread sticks made from Chebe Bread Mix.

Zesty Mac and Cheese

Make a box of GF macaroni and cheese, mix in a can of GF chili and heat through. Serve with carrot and celery sticks on the side.

Tacos

Ground beef or chicken tacos are great, as long as you make sure your taco seasoning, shredded cheddar cheese, and sour cream are all GF. Serve with lettuce, tomato, black olives, and GF salsa.

Burgers

Use ground beef to make your own hamburger patties and serve on Kinnik-Kwik Bread Buns. Make extra burgers and freeze them so you can take out one or two and grill them when needed. When you make Kinnik-Kwik Bread Buns, also make a few extra and freeze them for future use.

From Lila Brendel of Bismarck, North Dakota

Pasta Dinners

Pasta makes it easy to eat a creative gluten-free meal. Brown ground beef, add a GF pastas, and use your favorite seasonings, tomatoes, GF cheese, vegetables, or anything else you want to add. Plus, it only takes 20 minutes to prepare a meal!

Fajitas

Corn tortilla topped with cheese and your favorite meat, mushroom, onion, bell pepper, melted cheese, and GF salsa.

Great Summer Potatoes

Use potatoes and any other vegetables you like. Try potatoes (cut into cubes) with zucchini, carrots, green beans, bell peppers, onion, butter, seasoning salt, and pepper. Put ingredients in a 9- × 13-inch pan. Cover with about 2 Tbsp. butter and add about 1/2 cup water. Cover with foil and bake at 400 F. degrees for 30 minutes or until vegetables are tender.

From Marcy Thorner of New Market, Maryland

Keep things simple when preparing family meals. A grilled meat, rice or potatoes prepared your favorite way, steamed or stir-fried vegetables, and salad makes a simple, enjoyable meal that the whole family can enjoy and is healthy for all. A child with celiac disease who can eat whatever is on the table will feel less isolated.

From Rolf Meyersohn of New York City, New York

Polenta and Risotto

I use a microwave oven to make polenta from cornmeal, as well as risotto from Arborio rice, without having to stir endlessly. Barbara Kafka's *Microwave Gourmet* (William Morrow, 1998) has excellent recipes for these dishes as well as many others.

Chicken Stock

I make chicken stock every month or so, from bones collected and frozen from our roast chicken. Homemade chicken stock works well, especially in risotto, where salt-free (not to mention gluten-free) stock is needed. Cover chicken carcass and bones with water; add a carrot, celery stalk, an onion, a bay leaf, and peppercorns. Simmer for 90 minutes.

From Stacy Baran of Manchester, Maryland

Quick Chicken Quesadilla

My favorite lunch so far is to make quesadillas, using chopped Perdue Shortcuts Southwestern Style chicken, shredded Monterey jack Cheese, black beans, and onions layered between two corn tortillas. Microwave until it's warm and the cheese is melted, and it's an instant gluten-free quesadilla. It would also be great with GF salsa and sour cream on top!

My Favorite Smoothie

Mix a cup of vanilla yogurt, a cup of frozen mixed berries and small piece of banana, and blend in blender.

From Annie Hanaway of Portland, Oregon

My Favorite Hot Breakfast Cereal

My favorite hot breakfast cereal is what I call the "Trifecta." Put a total of 1/4 cup of whole grains in a bowl: 1/3 of this is amaranth, 1/3 is quinoa, and 1/3 is teff. Use 1 cup very hot water and a pinch of sea salt, then cook in microwave for 88 seconds at full power, then 15 minutes at power level 2. (You may have to experiment with the microwave power levels and cooking times.) It is really yummy!

Chapter 6

Delightful Gluten-Free Recipes

There are so many great gluten-free recipes to try and wonderful resources available to help you find these recipes. Look into cookbooks, Websites, newsletters, and message boards that can help (see Chapter 9). The following recipes can help you get started on your way to delicious gluten-free cooking.

Ham and Cheese Omelet With Fresh Basil

From Kit Kellison of Chesapeake, Virginia

Serve these omelets with hash browns, orange slices, and tomato juice.

1/4 cup chopped onion

1 oz. sharp white cheddar or Asiago cheese, shredded

2 thin slices GF deli ham, rolled and sliced into thin strips

3 eggs, well beaten

3-4 leaves fresh basil, chopped

1 Tbsp. butter or olive oil

Salt and pepper to taste

In an omelet pan (gluten-free Teflon or stainless steel), sauté onions on medium heat until they begin to brown and release a sweet aroma. Add the ham and cook until slightly brown. Add the basil and eggs, mixing in the cheese before the egg completely sets. This will make it a bit more quiche-like. Lift the mixture up off the pan occasionally to let the uncooked egg run to the bottom.

When the bottom is cooked well, flip the mixture over to cook the other side. It is important to use enough oil and not to let the pan get too hot to do this properly and to keep the egg from sticking to the pan. Fold the omelet on the plate and sprinkle some extra cheese in the middle and on top, if desired. Cover with a pot lid for five minutes to let the cheese melt and the flavors blend a bit before serving.

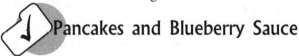 Pancakes and Blueberry Sauce

From Allan Gardyne's Website Best Gluten-Free Recipes (*http://members.ozemail.com.au/~coeliac/det.html*).

Serve with syrup and fruit juice.

Pancakes:

1 cup brown rice flour

1 cup white rice flour

1 1/4 cups water

2 eggs

Blend everything except the eggs in a food processor. Allow the mixture to stand for at least two hours. Add the eggs and beat. Brush a frying pan with oil. Pour in some of the mixture. Cover with a lid and cook on medium-low heat about 5 minutes. Turn with a spatula and cook the other side. Repeat.

Sauce:

1 oz. butter

1/4 cup blueberry jam

1/3 cup chicken stock (can use gluten-free stock cubes)

2 tsp. arrowroot

1/3 cup red wine

1 Tbsp. brown sugar

Melt butter and jam in a saucepan over low heat. Add stock, red wine, sugar, and arrowroot. Keeping it on a low heat, stir until the sauce thickens. Serve over pancakes.

Cheesy Potato and Ham Casserole

From Allan Gardyne's Website Best Gluten-Free Recipes (*http://members.ozemail.com.au/~coeliac/det.html*)

3 medium potatoes, peeled and thinly sliced

1 onion, sliced

2 hard-boiled eggs, chopped

3/4 cup GF cheese, grated

1/4 cup cooked GF ham, chopped

1/2 cup milk

2 Tbsp. GF chutney

1/4 tsp. paprika

Freshly ground black pepper

Herb salt

Grease an oven-safe dish. Add half the potato and onion slices. Sprinkle with salt and pepper. Spread the cheese, ham, chutney, and eggs over the potato slices. Pour half the milk over the mixture. Use the remaining potato and onion slices to make another layer. Add the remaining milk and sprinkle with paprika. Bake in 360-degree F. oven for about 30 minutes. The potatoes should be tender. If using a microwave, cook for 15 to 20 minutes.

Make-Ahead Brunch Casserole

From *Gluten-Free Cooking for Dummies* by Connie Sarros and Danna Korn (For Dummies, 2008)

Avoid the hassle of having to make all the food the morning of your brunch. Assemble this dish the day before, and just pop it in the oven before your friends arrive. Then sit back and listen to the raves!

This recipe is for a 9-inch-square dish, but you can easily double the ingredients to fit a 9- × 13-inch pan for a larger crowd.

Nonstick cooking spray

3 large Idaho potatoes, boiled, peeled, and diced

5 hard-boiled eggs, peeled and diced

3/4 pound low-salt GF ham, cut into 1/2-inch cubes

1/4 green pepper, minced

1/2 medium onion, minced

2 Tbsp. chopped fresh parsley

1/4 tsp. pepper

1 cup plus 2 Tbsp. sharp cheddar cheese, grated

2 Tbsp. butter, melted

2 1/2 Tbsp. cornstarch

8-ounce container sour cream

Paprika

Preheat oven to 375 degrees F. Lightly spray a 9-inch square baking dish with nonstick cooking spray. Place the diced potatoes, eggs, ham, green pepper, and onion in the baking dish. Sprinkle the parsley, pepper, and 1 cup of cheese on top; using a spoon, toss the ingredients lightly to distribute the cheese evenly. In a small bowl, stir together the melted butter, cornstarch, and sour cream (the mixture will be thick). Spoon tablespoonfuls of the mixture on top of the casserole. With the back of the spoon, smooth the topping to cover the casserole evenly. Sprinkle the top with the remaining cheese and paprika. Bake the casserole at 375 degrees F. for 35 minutes. Let the dish set for 5 minutes before serving. Serves 6.

Delicious Dining: Lunch and Dinner Recipes

Fast Beef Stroganoff

From Allan Gardyne's Website Best Gluten-Free Recipes (*http://members.ozemail.com.au/~coeliac/det.html*)

Serve over brown rice with steamed spinach

1/2 lb. ground beef

1 packet GF onion soup mix

3 cups GF rice noodles

1/2 tsp. ground ginger

3 1/2 cups hot water

1 can sliced mushrooms

1 cup cream

Maize corn flour or cornstarch

Microwave meat on high for 5 minutes. Add packet of soup, noodles, ginger, hot water. Cook 12 minutes. Add mushrooms and cream and thicken with maize corn flour. Microwave for another minute.

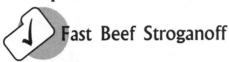Carol Fenster′s Pizza Crust & Pizza Sauce

From Carol Fenster, PhD, of Savory Palate, Inc. (*www.savorypalate.com*)

Serve with salad and gluten-free dressing

Pizza Sauce:

1 can (8 oz.) tomato sauce

1/2 tsp. dried oregano leaves

1/2 tsp. dried basil leaves

1/2 tsp. crushed dried rosemary

1/2 tsp. fennel seeds

1/4 tsp. garlic powder

2 tsp. sugar

1/2 tsp. salt

Combine all ingredients in small saucepan and bring to boil over medium heat. Reduce heat to low and simmer for 15 minutes, while pizza crust is being assembled. Makes about 1 cup.

Pizza Crust:

1 Tbsp. dry yeast

2/3 cup brown rice flour or garbanzo/fava bean flour

1/2 cup and 2 Tbsp. tapioca flour

2 tsp. xanthan gum*

1/2 tsp. salt

1 tsp. unflavored gelatin powder (Knox)

1 tsp. Italian herb seasoning

2/3 cup warm milk (110 degrees F.) or non-dairy liquid

1/2 tsp. sugar or honey

1 tsp. olive oil

1 tsp. cider vinegar

Extra rice flour for sprinkling

Preheat oven to 425 degrees F. In medium mixer bowl using regular beaters (not dough hooks), blend the yeast, flours, xanthan gum, salt, gelatin powder, and Italian seasoning on low speed. Add warm milk, sugar, oil, and vinegar. Beat on high speed for 2 minutes. (If the mixer bounces around the bowl, the dough is too stiff. Add water if necessary, 1 tablespoon at a time, until dough does not resist beaters.) The dough will resemble soft bread dough. (You may also mix in bread machine on dough setting.) Put mixture on lightly greased 12-inch pizza pan. Liberally sprinkle rice flour onto dough, then press dough into pan, continuing to sprinkle dough with flour to prevent sticking to your hands. Make edges thicker to hold the toppings.

Bake pizza crust for 10 minutes. Remove from oven. Top pizza crust with sauce, gluten-free cheese, and your preferred toppings. Bake for another 20–25 minutes or until top is nicely browned.

Serves 6 (1 slice per serving).

 Spaghetti Pie

From Connie Sarros, author of *Wheat-Free Gluten-free Cookbook for Kids and Busy Adults* **(McGraw-Hill, 2003)**

Serve with tossed salad and gluten-free dressing.

1 Tbsp. olive oil

4 cups cooked, GF spaghetti (about 1/2 lb. uncooked)

2 cups GF spaghetti sauce

1/2 cup GF Parmesan cheese, grated

1/4 tsp. red pepper flakes

1/2 tsp. basil

3/4 tsp. oregano

1/4 tsp. garlic powder

1 Tbsp. parsley flakes

1/2 cup GF mozzarella cheese, grated

Preheat oven to 350 degrees F. Pour oil into a 9-inch pie plate.

Use a pastry brush to spread it on the bottom and sides of the pan. Put spaghetti into a large bowl. Use a clean pair of scissors to cut it into smaller pieces. Pour the spaghetti sauce over the spaghetti. Sprinkle the Parmesan cheese, red pepper flakes, basil, oregano, garlic powder, and parsley over the spaghetti.

Stir spaghetti with a fork to mix thoroughly. Pour spaghetti into pie plate. With the back of a spoon, pat it down. Sprinkle top with mozzarella cheese. Bake for 30 minutes. Cut the "pie" into wedges to serve.

Serves 6.

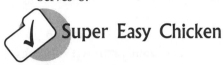

Super Easy Chicken

From Connie Sarros, author of *Wheat-Free Gluten-free Cookbook for Kids and Busy Adults* (McGraw-Hill, 2003)

1 Tbsp. light brown sugar

2 Tbsp. GF ketchup

3/4 cup GF salsa

4 boneless skinless chicken breast halves

Preheat oven to 400 degrees F. In a small bowl, stir together the brown sugar, salsa, and ketchup. Lay the chicken pieces in an 8-x-12 baking pan that has been sprayed with gluten-free, non-stick spray. Spoon the salsa mixture over the chicken pieces. Let the chicken marinate at room temperature for 20 minutes. Bake for 40 minutes or until the chicken is cooked through.

Serves 4.

Almost Cheeseburger

From Connie Sarros, author of *Wheat-Free Gluten-free Cookbook for Kids and Busy Adults* (McGraw-Hill, 2003)

1/2 lb. lean ground beef

1 tsp. dried minced onion flakes

1 lb. GF processed cheese, cut into cubes

1/4 cup milk

2 Tbsp. GF ketchup

2 Tbsp. GF mustard

Brown the beef and onion flakes in a skillet that has been sprayed with a gluten-free nonstick spray, breaking up the meat with a fork as it cooks. Stir in the cheese, milk, ketchup, and mustard; stir until the cheese has melted. Use as a dip with crackers, as a "cheeseburger" with gluten-free bread "fingers" as dippers, or as a main meal by serving it over boiled, gluten-free elbow macaroni.

Yields 4 cups. Serving size: 1/2 cup.

 ## Mexican Lasagna

From Clare Popowich of Belchertown, Massachusetts

1 lb. ground beef or turkey

1 pkg. GF taco seasoning mix

1 can GF refried beans

1 can GF tomato sauce or salsa

1 pkg. corn tortillas

1 pkg. shredded cheddar cheese

Prepare beef and taco seasoning mix according to package directions. Mix refried beans and tomato sauce or salsa, reserving about 1/2 cup of sauce or salsa for the top. Spread a little bean mixture into casserole to keep tortillas from sticking. Layer tortillas, bean mixture, and cheese, ending with tortillas. Spread with reserved tomato sauce/salsa and sprinkle with cheese. Bake at 350 degrees F. until bubbly. This can be prepared ahead of time and reheats well. (If you prefer your dishes cheesier or saucier, increase ingredients accordingly.) Serve with taco condiments.

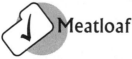 ## Meatloaf

From Clan Thompson (*www.clanthompson.com*)

1 cup GF bread crumbs

1 onion, chopped and lightly fried

1 egg, slightly beaten

1 Tbsp. GF soy sauce

3/4 tsp. dry mustard

1/4 tsp. garlic powder

1/4 tsp. salt

1/4 tsp. black pepper

1/4 cup milk

1 lb. ground beef

Mix all the ingredients together in a large bowl. Place into a greased pan. Bake in a preheated 350-degree F. oven for about one hour. If you want leftovers for meatloaf sandwiches, you may want to double the amounts!

 # My Favorite Pie Crust

From Clan Thompson (*www.clanthompson.com*)

2/3 cup cornstarch

2/3 cup soy flour

2/3 cup tapioca flour

1 tsp. baking powder

1 tsp. xanthan gum

1 tsp. salt

1 Tbsp. white sugar

2/3 cup Crisco

1 egg

5 Tbsp. cold water

Cornstarch for rolling

Put the flour, baking powder, xanthan gum, salt, and sugar into a medium bowl. Cut in the Crisco until you have small pieces the size of lima beans. Mix the egg and the 5 tablespoons cold water in a separate cup. Add 5 tablespoons of this mixture to the flour and stir well. If necessary, add more liquid until the dough forms into a ball. Refrigerate at least an hour to chill.

Divide the dough in half. Roll the first half out onto a board dusted with cornstarch. Transfer to a pie tin. If the crust breaks, just piece it together in the pie tin and press the dough back together. Fill the crust with appropriate filling. Use the remainder of the dough to cut strips for a lattice crust. Cook at 350 degrees F. or as recipe for filling directs. Makes enough crust for one two-crust pie.

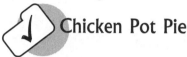 ## Chicken Pot Pie

From Clan Thompson (*www.clanthompson.com*)
For the crust, use the My Favorite Pie Crust recipe on page 116.
Filling:
6 Tbsp. butter
6 Tbsp. cornstarch
3 cups milk
1 tsp. salt
1/4 tsp. black pepper
1/4 tsp. crushed garlic
16-oz. package frozen vegetables
4–6 chicken thighs, cooked, or an equivalent amount of breast or leg meat

Melt butter in a heavy-bottomed saucepan over low heat. Slowly add cornstarch and blend well. Gradually add milk, blending well. Continue to stir as the sauce thickens. Bring to a boil and reduce heat, stirring for another 2–3 minutes. Remove from heat. Add salt, black pepper, and crushed garlic. Add one 14- to16-oz. package of frozen vegetables, preferably the Bird's Eye combination that includes pea pods, carrots, peas, and baby corn. Add the chicken. Place the bottom crust in a 8- or 9-inch pie pan. Fill pan with the chicken, vegetables, and sauce. Make a lattice crust to cover the pie. Cook at 350 degrees F. for 45 minutes or until done.

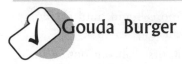

Gouda Burger

Recipe from *www.glutenfreeda.com.*

Serve with gluten-free tortilla chips and gluten-free salsa.

1/2 lb. ground beef

1 shallot, minced

2 tsp. Worcestershire sauce

Salt and freshly ground black pepper

1 large garlic clove, minced and divided

2 Shiitake mushrooms, sliced

1 Tbsp. olive oil, divided

2 1/4-inch slices of a beefsteak tomato

1/2 cup mixed salad greens

1/4 cup sliced Gouda cheese

Herbed mayonnaise (see page 119)

In a large bowl, combine the ground beef, shallot, 1/2 of the minced garlic, and Worcestershire sauce. Form hamburger mixture into 2 1/2-inch thick patties. Season patties with salt and freshly ground black pepper. Set aside.

In a small skillet, heat 1/2 Tbsp. of olive oil over medium heat. Add the remaining garlic and sauté for 30 seconds. Add the mushrooms and sauté for 3–4 minutes or until the mushrooms are tender and lightly browned. Remove from heat and set aside. Heat the remaining 1/2 Tbsp. of olive oil in a large skillet over medium-high heat. Add the hamburger patties and cook for 4 minutes per side, or until nicely browned on both sides and cooked through.

To assemble the burger, place the beefsteak tomato slice in the center of a plate. Top the tomato with a hamburger patty and spread 1 heaping Tbsp. of the herbed mayonnaise on top of the burger. Top with 1/2 the cheese and 1/2 the sautéed mushrooms. Garnish the top of the burger with mixed greens. Repeat assembly with remaining burger. Serve immediately.

Makes 2 servings.

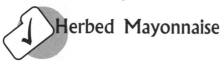

Herbed Mayonnaise

1/4 cup GF mayonnaise
2 tsp. Italian parsley, chopped
1 Tbsp. fresh basil, chopped
Combine in a small bowl.

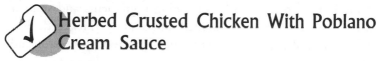

Herbed Crusted Chicken With Poblano Cream Sauce

From *www.glutenfreeda.com.*

4 chicken quarters
2 Tbsp. cumin seeds
1/2 tsp. chipotle powder or chili powder
2 Tbsp. roasted garlic, chopped
2 tsp. salt
2 tsp. peppercorns, crushed
2 Tbsp. olive oil

Preheat oven to 375 degrees F. In a small bowl, combine cumin seeds, chipotle powder, garlic, salt, crushed peppercorns, and olive oil. Rub generously over washed and dried chicken pieces.

Place chicken in a baking dish and bake for 1 hour and 20 minutes (or 80 minutes). After 45 minutes, remove chicken from oven and baste with pan juices and continue basting every 15 minutes until done.

Poblano cream sauce:

2 Tbsp. olive oil

1 poblano chile, chopped

3/4 cup onion, chopped

4 cloves garlic, minced

3/4 cup cilantro, chopped

1/4 cup whipping cream

1/2 cup crème fraiche, or GF sour cream

Salt and pepper to taste

Heat oil in a heavy saucepan over medium heat. Add chile and onion and sauté until onion is just translucent. Add garlic and sauté for 1 more minute. Add remaining ingredients and simmer for 2 minutes until sauce is blended and slightly thickened. Season with salt and pepper. Transfer sauce to a food processor and process until smooth.

Remove chicken from oven and spoon a layer of sauce on tops of chicken quarters. Return to oven for 10 minutes. Serve immediately.

Makes 4 servings.

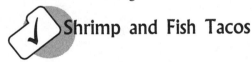

Shrimp and Fish Tacos

From *www.glutenfreeda.com.*

This recipe takes a bit of prep but is well worth the effort. Instead of broiling the fish and shrimp, you can grill them if you prefer.

Serve with gluten-free Mexican rice and gluten-free mayonnaise.

Tacos:

6 Tbsp. ground dried New Mexico or California chilies, or 1–2 tsp. red pepper flakes

3 Tbsp. salad oil

1/2 tsp. pepper

1/2 tsp. salt

1/2 tsp. garlic powder

1/2 tsp. cayenne

1/2 tsp. ground cumin

2 whole cloves

1 dried bay leaf, broken into pieces

3/4 lb. boned, fresh skinned firm-flesh fish such as halibut or mahi-mahi

1/2 lb. medium size prawns, peeled and deveined

1/4 cabbage, sliced thin

12 GF corn tortillas

In a large bowl, mix ground dried chilies, oil, pepper, 1/2 tsp. salt, garlic powder, cayenne, cumin, cloves, and bay leaf. Rinse fish and shrimp; pat dry. Add to bowl and turn to coat with marinade; cover and chill at least 1 hour or up to 1 day, mixing several times.

Pico de Gallo:

2 cups diced tomatoes

1/2 cup finely diced onion

2 Tbsp. minced jalapeño chili

1/4 cup minced fresh cilantro

2 Tbsp. lime juice

1 garlic clove, minced

Salt to taste

In a bowl, combine all ingredients. Salt to taste.

Cilantro-Jalapeño Mayonnaise:

1 3/4 cup GF mayonnaise (see recipe on page 122)

2 Tbsp. water

2 Tbsp. cider vinegar

1 jalapeño chili

1 garlic clove

1/2 cup lightly packed cilantro

1/4 teaspoon pepper

Salt to taste

In a blender or food processor, combine all ingredients. Whirl until smooth. Add salt to taste.

Heat tortillas one at a time over medium high heat in a heavy skillet. Keep warm by wrapping in foil. Lift fish from marinade and arrange pieces in a single layer in a 9- x 13-inch pan. Discard marinade. Broil fish 4–5 inches from heat until opaque but still moist-looking in center of thickest part (cut to test), about 5 minutes for 1/2 inch thick pieces. With a slotted spatula, transfer fish to towels to blot oil, then set on a platter. Cut fish along the grain into 1/2-inch slices and shrimp into 1/2-inch pieces; season to taste with salt.

To assemble tacos:

Spread a layer of cilantro-jalapeño mayonnaise on a heated tortilla, top with fish and shrimp mixture, cabbage, and pico de gallo.

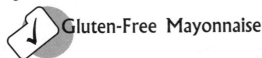

Gluten-Free Mayonnaise

From *www.glutenfreeda.com*

For perfect results every time, use a food processor with an attachment that allows liquid to be added in a very small stream. Fill with oil and process while oil is added very slowly.

1 whole egg

1 tsp. GF stone-ground mustard

1 Tbsp. lemon juice

1/2 tsp. salt

Fresh ground white pepper

Dash of cayenne

1 cup vegetable oil

Add all the ingredients to a food processor or blender except the oil. Blend briefly. With the motor running add the oil in a slow, thin, steady stream. After the mayonnaise is made, correct the seasoning to taste.

Makes 4 servings.

Italian Bacon and Tomato Risotto

From Stacy LaRoche of New York, New York

1/2 lb. sliced bacon

1 onion, chopped

Few handfuls of cherry tomatoes, halved

14 oz. GF chicken broth

1/2 cup of milk or milk substitute

1 tsp. dried parsley

2 cups instant rice

1/2 cup grated cheese

Cook sliced bacon and chopped onion in a skillet. Drain. Stir in halved cherry tomatoes, chicken broth, milk, dried parsley, and instant rice. Bring to a boil over medium heat. Simmer for 5 minutes over low heat. Add grated cheese to taste. Let stand 5 minutes. Serve topped with grated cheese.

This is very fast if you have a pressure cooker and use real risotto, which I prefer. If you don't have a pressure cooker, use instant rice, as directed. A pressure cooker will cook up real risotto in about the same amount of time as it takes to make instant rice and has a great deal more flavor.

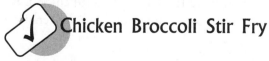Chicken Broccoli Stir Fry

From Jessica Duvall of Williamsburg, Kansas

1 lb boneless, skinless chicken breast

Few Tbsp. of cooking oil

1/3 cup GF soy sauce

Few cloves garlic, minced

1 1/2 cups water

2 cups broccoli

2 cups instant brown rice

Cut the chicken breast into chunks or strips and cook in oil until cooked through. Add soy sauce, garlic, and water; and bring to a boil. Stir in broccoli and instant brown rice. Cover and cook over low heat for approximately 5 minutes or until rice is done.

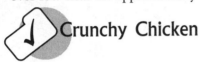Crunchy Chicken

From Kit Kellison of Chesapeake, Virginia

GF cooking spray

2 Tbsp. milk

1 egg, beaten

6 pieces chicken

1 cup GF cornflakes, crushed

2 Tbsp. butter

Salt

Black pepper

Prepare a shallow baking dish with cooking spray, and preheat oven to 400 degrees F. Mix milk and beaten egg. Dunk pieces chicken in egg mixture, salt and pepper both sides, and roll in crushed cornflake crumbs. Salt and pepper again, place on baking dish, and dot with butter. Bake for 1 hour or until chicken is cooked through. The chicken comes out moist, tender, crispy, and delicious!

Creamed Potatoes and Vegetables

From Lila Brendel of Bismarck, North Dakota
5–6 potatoes
1 bag frozen carrots, broccoli, and cauliflower mix
1/2 cup water
1 pint whipping cream
Salt
Black pepper

Cut up potatoes and place potatoes in large frying pan. Add salt, pepper and water and cook until almost tender, stirring frequently. Add vegetables and cream, and cook until cream bubbles and vegetables are hot.

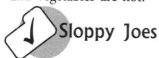 ## Sloppy Joes

From Joyce Etheridge of Avon, Indiana
1 lb. ground beef
3–4 Tbsp. brown sugar
1/2 onion, chopped
1 cup Muir Glen Organic Ketchup

Cook ground beef, onion, sugar and ketchup together in a frying pan. Spoon the mixture on gluten-free buns. Serve with salad and vegetables or potatoes.

 ## Quick and Delicious Pizza

From Ashley Cooper of Urbandale, Iowa
1 Kinnikinnick pizza crust
2 Tbsp. virgin olive oil
2 cloves garlic, minced

1 cup low-fat mozzarella cheese, shredded

2 tomatoes, sliced

Cut up mushrooms

Spread the olive oil and garlic on the pizza crust. Add your tomato slices and mushrooms. Cover with mozzarella cheese. Bake at 350 degrees F. for 15 minutes.

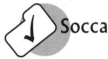 ## Socca

From Rolf Meyersohn of New York, New York

2/3 cup chickpea flour

4 Tbsp. olive oil

1/4 tsp. salt

1 cup water

Ground pepper to taste

Mix chickpea flour, 3 tablespoons olive oil. salt, water, and ground pepper and let rest 1 hour or more at room temp or in refrigerator. Preheat oven to 400 degrees F. Oil a round, shallow, nonstick pan and pour on batter, about 1/8 inch thick. Put under a moderate broiler as close to flame as possible. After 5 minutes, remaining olive oil on top and broil for 5–10 minutes more until crisp and golden, with the consistency of a thick crepe. Slide onto serving plate and cut into 2-inch wedges.

All-in-One Crock-Pot Recipes

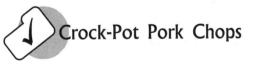 ## Crock-Pot Pork Chops

From Connie Sarros, author of *Wheat-Free Gluten-free Cookbook for Kids and Busy Adults* (McGraw-Hill, 2003)

Serve with gluten-free au gratin potatoes and steamed cauliflower.

1 lb. pork chops

1/2 tsp. garlic powder

3 Tbsp. GF soy sauce

1/2 cup GF Italian dressing

1 small bottle GF barbecue sauce

Wash pork chops under cold running water. Pat dry with paper towels. Sprinkle garlic powder on both sides of chops. Place chops in a large self-seal plastic bag. Pour the soy sauce and the Italian dressing into bag. Seal bag securely. Move bag around to distribute the dressing between the chops. Refrigerate bag several hours.

Remove pork chops from the marinade and place in a Crock-Pot. Pour the barbecue sauce over the chops, lifting the chops with a fork to distribute the sauce evenly. Cover Crock-Pot and cook on low for 8 hours.

Serves 6.

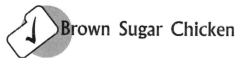Brown Sugar Chicken

From Stephanie O'Dea of *www.crockpot365.blogspot.com.*

12 boneless, skinless chicken thighs, or 6 boneless, skinless breast halves

1 cup brown sugar

1/4 cup lemon-lime soda

2/3 cup white wine vinegar

3 cloves smashed and chopped garlic

2 Tbsp. soy sauce (La Choy and Tamari Wheat Free are GF)

1 tsp. ground black pepper

Use a 5-6 quart Crock-Pot for this recipe.

Place the chicken in your Crock-Pot. Cover with the brown sugar, pepper, chopped garlic, and soy sauce. Add the vinegar and pour in the soda. It will bubble! Cover and cook on low for 6-9 hours, or on high for 4-5 hours. The chicken is done when it is cooked through and has reached desired consistency. The longer you cook it, the more tender it will be.

Serve over a bowl of white or brown rice with a ladle full of the broth.

Creamy White Bean and Apple Chili

From Stephanie O'Dea of *www.crockpot365.blogspot.com*.

2 15-oz. cans of white beans, drained and rinsed

1 onion, chopped

2 apples, cut in tiny chunks

3 cloves smashed and chopped garlic

3 Tbsp. butter

2 tsp. chili powder

1/2 tsp. ground thyme

1 tsp. cumin

1/4 tsp. salt

1/4 tsp. pepper

3 cups chicken broth

1/2 cup plain nonfat yogurt

1/2 cup sharp cheddar cheese, shredded (optional)

Any Crock-Pot over 4 quarts would work well with this dish. Put the butter into the bottom of your Crock-Pot. Pour in the drained and rinsed beans, onion, and apple. Add the spices, and pour in the broth. Stir in the yogurt. Cover and cook on low for 8 hours, or on high for 4-5 hours. This is done when the onion has reached desired tenderness and the flavors have melded. Stir in the cheddar cheese before serving.

Lighten It Up: Soups and Salads

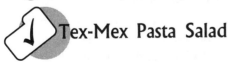

Tex-Mex Pasta Salad

From The Gluten-Free Pantry (*www.glutenfree.com*).

1 10-oz. package gluten-free fusilli or elbow rice pasta

1 14.5-oz. can black beans, rinsed and drained

1 cup frozen corn kernels, thawed

1 red bell pepper, seeded and chopped

3 green onions, chopped

1 cup cooked chicken, cubed (optional)

1 cup GF medium salsa (check labels)

1/2 cup GF plain yogurt or GF low-fat sour cream

3 Tbsp. GF mayonnaise

2 tsp. ground cumin

Salt and pepper to taste

Cook pasta, drain, and rinse in cold water. Combine drained pasta, black beans, corn, pepper, green onions, and chicken, (if used). In a separate bowl, combine salsa, yogurt or sour cream, mayonnaise, cumin, and salt and pepper. Pour over pasta mixture and stir to blend. Refrigerate until ready to serve.

Serves 8.

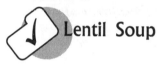

Lentil Soup

From Clan Thompson of *www.clanthompson.com.*

1 1/2 Tbsp. oil

1 large onion

1 clove garlic

1/3 cup brown rice

2 cups dried lentils, washed and picked over

2 quarts cold water

1 hambone with meat

2 potatoes, peeled and cut

2 carrots, sliced

1 large rib of celery, chopped

1/4 cup (scant) celery leaves, chopped

1 cup tomato juice

1 tsp. dried basil

2 Tbsp. chopped fresh parsley or 2 tsp. dried parsley

1/2 cup dry white wine

Salt and pepper to taste

Cook the onion, garlic, and brown rice in a pot in the oil for 5 minutes over low heat. Add lentils, 2 quarts cold water, and the hambone. Bring to a boil and cook 1 hour. Add potatoes, carrots, celery rib and leaves, tomato juice, basil, parsley, salt, and pepper. Cook for 30 to 60 minutes, until vegetables are tender. Cut meat off bone and remove bone. Stir in 1/2 cup of dry white wine and serve. Replenish water while cooking as needed.

Serves 10–12.

Betsy's Creamy Potato Cauliflower Soup

From The Gluten-free Pantry (*www.glutenfree.com*)

Serve with tossed salad and Yummy Breadstick.

1 1/2 cups potatoes peeled and diced

2 small celery sticks, diced

1 small onion, minced

1 1/2 cups water

1 1/2 cups cauliflower in small florets, steamed for 5 minutes

1 tsp. salt

Cook everything but the cauliflower until tender. Mash (do not drain). Add cauliflower.

White sauce:

2 Tbsp. butter

1 1/2 cups milk or milk substitute

2 Tbsp. cornstarch

Bring white sauce ingredients to a boil and stir continuously until mixture thickens. Fold into soup. Garnish with parsley and serve. Serves 4.

Jazz It Up: Sauce

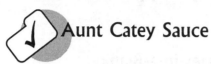 Aunt Catey Sauce

From Tim Coda of Salt Lake City, Utah

This recipe is named after my great Aunt Catey. She always seemed to have this on hand on the farm in Illinois. My father used to say, "This would even make shoe laces edible."

3 Tbsp. butter

1 Tbsp. peanut oil (or substitute more butter)

3/4 cup onion, diced finely

3–5 cloves garlic, minced

3 cups milk

1–1 1/2 cups Velveeta cheese, in 1/2-inch cubes

pinch salt and pepper

1 tsp. basil

1/4 cup white wine (optional)

2–3 Tbsp. corn starch dissolved in equal amount cold water

In saucepan, sauté garlic and onions in butter and oil. Add milk, wine, and seasonings and heat on low for 5 to 10 minutes. Slowly add cheese, stirring constantly as it will scorch to the bottom of the pan until just about to boil. When just beginning to boil, thicken with cornstarch mixture.

Serve over vegetables or gluten-free pasta.

Be the Life of the Party: Appetizers and Party Foods

 Chebe Bread Piggies-in-a-Blanket

From Regina Celano of Ronkonkoma, New York

1 cup GF cheese, shredded

2 eggs

2 Tbsp. oil

1/3 cup water

20 GF cocktail franks or GF sausages

Using a bread dough mixer, or with a spoon, blend cheese, eggs, oil, and water. Mix well with hands for 5 minutes or until very smooth and well-blended. (Add a little water if too dry; add Chebe mix or food starch if too sticky.) Roll into 20 balls and flatten each one. Place a cocktail frank or sausage on each piece of dough and roll them up. Place on non-greased baking sheet and bake at 375 degrees F. until golden brown.

 White Sauce/Salsa-Cheese Dip

From Kit Kellison of Chesapeake, Virginia

2 Tbsp. butter

1 Tbsp. potato flour

1 cup milk

4 ounces Kraft mild cheddar cheese, shredded (check label)

1 Tbsp. GF salsa

Make a roux by melting butter over medium heat and stirring in the potato flour until it starts to bubble. Turn up heat a bit and slowly add milk until it thins the roux into the texture of a set pudding. Thin a little more and then stir for a couple of minutes to allow the flour to cook and to make sure the mixture doesn't get too thick. Add more milk as needed and monitor the heat.

If you have gotten this far, you have just made a white sauce that can be adapted to make any other milk gravy, cream sauce, or soup you would like. When the sauce is at milk-gravy consistency, stir in 1 ounce of the cheese at a time, stirring in between until it is all blended and melted. At this point you might want to taste the mixture to see if it is cheesy enough. You may add more cheese if you prefer, incorporating it in slowly, mixing all the while. When the mixture is smooth, add the salsa, which will bring the color up and add a nice tang.

Serve with heated tortilla chips.

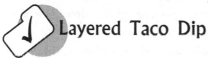

Layered Taco Dip

From Regina Celano of Ronkonkoma, New York

1 8-oz. package GF cream cheese, shoften
1 8-oz. package of GF cheddar cheese, shredded
1 can of Hormel chili with beans
1 16-oz. bag of GF tortilla chips

In a microwave-safe 8- x 8-inch pan spread the softened cream cheese, top with the contents of the can of chili, and pour the bag of shredded cheddar over the chili. Microwave until the cheese gets bubbly. Dip the tortilla chips and enjoy!

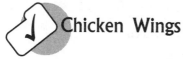

Chicken Wings

From Lila Brendel of Bismarck, North Dakota

4 lbs. chicken wings or drumsticks
1 cup GF soy sauce
1 cup water
1/4 cup oil

1/2 cup pineapple juice

1 tsp. ginger

1 tsp. garlic

1 cup sugar

Mix ingredients and marinate chicken overnight. Bake on cookie sheet at 350 degrees F. for 90 minutes.

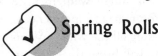 ## Spring Rolls

From *Recipes for Special Diets* by Connie Sarros (*http:// gfbooks.homestead.com*)

The ingredients are dairy-free, egg-free, gluten-free, low sodium, peanut- and tree-nut-free, and approved for diabetics.

For corn-free diets, use arrowroot or potato flour in place of cornstarch.

For soy-free diets, omit the soy sauce.

For yeast-free diets, omit the sherry.

For vegetarian and vegan diets, add 1/4 cup chopped green pepper and 1/4 cup chopped bamboo shoots in place of the shrimp.

1 Tbsp. cornstarch

2 Tbsp. dry sherry

2 Tbsp. GF soy sauce

1/4 tsp. sugar

1/4 tsp. dry ginger

2 Tbsp. sesame oil

2 cups packed napa cabbage, finely-sliced

1/3 cup green onions, sliced thin

1/2 cup mushrooms, chopped

3 cans (4 ounces each) small shrimp, drained

1/2 cup bean sprouts, chopped

36 GF rice papers

Mix first 5 ingredients in a cup; set aside. Heat 1 Tbsp. sesame oil in a large skillet. Add cabbage, onions, and mushrooms; stir-fry for 2 minutes. Stir in shrimp and bean sprouts. Pour in soy sauce mixture and heat, stirring constantly, until thickened. Remove pan from heat. Soak rice papers in water for 3 minutes to soften. Lay one rice paper a flat surface. Place 1 heaping Tbsp. filling at one edge of the paper. Roll paper, folding in sides, to form a cylinder. Place roll on a greased baking sheet. Repeat with remaining rolls. Brush tops of rolls lightly with remaining 1 Tbsp. sesame oil. Bake at 375 degrees F. for 15 minutes until tops are crisp.

Serve hot. (When rice papers cool after being baked, they tend to get rubbery.) Makes 36 spring rolls.

Everyone's Favorites: Desserts and Breads

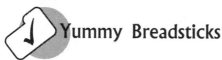

Yummy Breadsticks

From The Gluten-Free Pantry (*www.glutenfree.com*)

1 bag Bagel Mix from The Gluten-Free Pantry

1 tsp. salt

3 Tbsp. grated Parmesan cheese

1 Tbsp. GF yeast

1–2 tsp. dry basil

1–2 tsp. dry oregano

1 egg plus 1 egg white, lightly beaten

2 Tbsp. olive oil

1 cup warm water

2 Tbsp. honey

1 tsp. cider vinegar

1 egg yolk plus 1 Tbsp. warm water to brush breadsticks

Preheat oven to 425 degrees F.

Combine the Bagel Mix with the rest of the dry ingredients in a bowl. Mix all the wet ingredients together in a separate bowl. Beat liquids into dry ingredients using a heavy-duty mixer. Beat for two to three minutes or until mixture is smooth. Roll into 10 9-inch lengths between layers of oiled plastic wrap. Transfer to breadstick pan or baking sheets. Cover with oiled plastic wrap and let rise 30–40 minutes.

Brush with beaten egg yolk mixture and sprinkle with coarse salt. Bake 16–18 minutes. Cool slightly before serving.

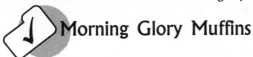 # Morning Glory Muffins

From Annie Hanaway of Portland, Oregon

1/2 cup raisins

1/2 cup potato flour

1/4 cup soy flour

1/8 cup garfava flour

1/2 cup brown sugar

2 tsp. cinnamon

1 cup grated carrot

1 large tart apple, grated

1/2 cup walnuts, chopped

3 eggs

2 tsp. vanilla extract

1/2 cup brown rice flour

1/4 cup tapioca flour

1/4 cup sorghum flour

1/8 cup rice bran

2 tsp. baking powder

1/2 tsp. salt

1 cup grated zucchini

1/2 cup shredded unsweetened coconut

1/2 tsp. grated ginger

2/3 cup oil: coconut, walnut, or almond

Preheat oven to 400 degrees F. Use parchment papers to line muffin tins.

Cover raisins with hot water and soak while making rest of recipe. Stir together the flours, sugar, baking soda, cinnamon and salt. Mix thoroughly to integrate the different flours. In a medium bowl, combine carrot, apple, zucchini, coconut, walnuts, and ginger, and mix well. Stir into flour and mix thoroughly. In a small bowl, whisk eggs and beat in oils and vanilla. Make a well in the center of the dry ingedients and pour in egg-oil mixture. Drain raisins and add in, stirring batter gently until fully mixed. Spoon into muffin tins and bake approximately 20 minutes. Makes about 16 muffins.

 ## Harvest Pumpkin Bread/Cupcakes/Muffins

From Connie Rieper of Fayetteville, Arkansas

1 cup brown sugar

1/3 cup butter, softened, or cooking oil

1/2 tsp. GF vanilla extract

2 eggs

1 can pumpkin

1/4 cup milk (use soy milk or juice if you have other food intolerances)

1 cup flour mix (use white rice, potato starch, tapioca, xanthan gum)

1/2 tsp. salt

1/2 tsp. ginger

1/2 tsp. nutmeg

1/4 tsp. ground clove

2 tsp. cinnamon

1 1/2 tsp. baking powder

Preheat oven to 250–275 degrees F.

Grease pans. In large bowl, cream butter and sugar with mixer. Add vanilla, eggs, pumpkin, and milk in order. Mix well.

Mix all dry ingredients together. Add to the large bowl. Blend wet and dry ingredients together. Add walnuts and raisins. Pour into cupcake, muffin, or bread pans. Bake small cupcakes/muffins for 20 minutes, larger cupcakes/muffins for 30 minutes, and bread for 40 minutes. They are done when a skewer inserted into the center comes out clean. Cooking times may vary with different ovens. When cooled, frost the cupcakes with gluten-free frosting.

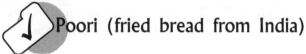

Poori (fried bread from India)

From Connie Rieper of Fayetteville, Arkansas

1 cup GF flour mix (or white rice flour)

1/2 tsp. salt

2 Tbsp. vegetable oil (for dough)

7–10 Tbsp. milk or water

3–4 cups vegetable oil (for frying)

Pour flour in bowl. Add salt and mix. Dribble oil over the top and rub it into the flour with your fingers. Slowly (1 Tbsp. at a time) add milk or water, to form a medium-soft ball. Knead for 10 minutes, or until smooth. It should have consistency of new play-dough: no dry cracks, but not soggy or slimy. Form big ball, cover with oil, and let rest. Divide dough into 12 balls. Roll one ball out into about a 2- or 3-inch round . You can also cut a plastic baggie into two squares and roll the dough in between or flatten between your two hands.

Use a deep frying pan or wok and set over medium high heat. When oil is very hot, lay poori carefully on surface of oil, without letting it fold up. It should sizzle immediately (if it doesn't, heat oil more). Spoon hot oil over poori or dunk it under with a spoon with quick strokes. It should puff up in seconds. Turn poori over and cook for a few seconds. Remove with slotted spoon and place on paper towels. Serve immediately.

Lime Meringue Pie

From Clan Thompson (*www.clanthompson.com*)

1 1/2 cups sugar

5 Tbsp. cornstarch

1/8 tsp. salt

1 1/2 cups hot water

2 egg yolks, slightly beaten

Rind of 1/2 lime, grated

2 Tbsp. butter

1/3 cup lime juice

1 8- or 9-inch pastry shell (pre-baked and gluten-free)

2 egg whites

1 tsp. lime juice

6 Tbsp. sugar

Mix 1 1/2 cups of sugar, cornstarch, and salt in a saucepan. Blend in the hot water, gradually. Bring to a boil over high heat, stirring constantly. Reduce heat to medium. Cook and stir for 6 more minutes. Remove from heat. Stir a small amount of the hot mixture into the egg yolks and then add to the rest of the hot mixture. Bring to a boil over high heat, stirring constantly. Reduce heat to low and cook and stir constantly for 4 more minutes. Remove from heat. Add lime peel and butter. Stir in 1/3 cup lime juice. Cover surface with clear plastic wrap and cool for 10 minutes. Pour into your favorite pre-baked gluten-free pastry shell. Cool to room temperature.

To make meringue:

Beat egg whites with 1 tsp. lime juice until soft peaks form. Gradually add 6 Tbsp. sugar, beating until stiff peaks are formed. Spread meringue over the pie, making sure to seal to edges of pastry. Bake in a moderate oven (350 degrees F.) for 12–15 minutes or until the meringue is golden. Cool thoroughly before serving.

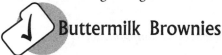

Buttermilk Brownies

From Jan Hammer of Fargo, North Dakota

Wet Mix:

1/2 cup oil

1/2 cup buttermilk

1/2 cup margarine

1 tsp. baking soda

1 cup cold water

2 eggs

2 cups sugar

2 1/4 cup flour mix (see below)

4 Tbsp. cocoa

Bring water, margarine, and oil to a boil. Add baking soda to buttermilk. Pour over dry ingredients. Beat until creamy. Add buttermilk, soda, and eggs. Beat well. Bake in 15- × 10-inch jelly-roll pan for 18 minutes at 400 degrees F.

Dry Flour Mix:

2 cups brown rice flour

2 cups white rice flour

1 1/2 cup sweet rice flour

2/3 cup cornstarch

1 1/3 cup tapioca starch or flour

1/2 cup rice bran or rice polish

2 tsp. xanthan gum

Sift all ingredients three or four times and store in canister. Use 1 cup of this mixture when recipe calls for 1 cup wheat flour. Works very well in cookies, bars, cakes—even rolled out sugar cookies.

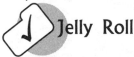 ## Jelly Roll

From Jean Wright of Allegany, New York

1 cup GF flour mixture (see page 142)

1 tsp. baking powder

1/4 tsp. salt

3 large eggs (3/4 cup)

1 cup sugar

1/3 cup water

1 tsp. vanilla

1/2 cup confectioner's sugar

Pre-heat oven to 375 degrees F. Grease a jelly roll pan (15- × 10-inch) and line bottom with greased parchment paper or greased aluminum foil. Blend flour, baking powder, and salt; set aside. Beat eggs in small mixing bowl until very thick and a light lemon color. (It takes a while!) Pour beaten eggs into large bowl. Gradually beat in sugar. Blend in water and vanilla, on low speed. Slowly mix in dry ingredients (low speed) until batter is smooth. Pour into pan. Bake 12 to 15 minutes. Loosen edges and immediately turn upside down on a towel sprinkled with half of the confectioner's sugar.

Remove paper. Trim stiff edges. While hot, roll cake and towel starting with the narrow end. Cool on wire rack. Unroll cake, remove towel. Spread with soft (not syrupy) jelly or filling of your choice. Roll again. Sprinkle with confectioner's sugar. Cut in 1-inch slices. You can cut it into 4 pieces widthwise and stack with filling (such as fresh strawberries, clear orange or lemon filling, or pudding) and top with whipped cream. If you want a chocolate roll just add 1/4 cup cocoa to dry ingredients.

Gluten-Free Flour Mixture

2 cups GF garbanzo and fava flour

3 cups tapioca flour

2 slightly rounded tsp. xanthan gum

1 cup GF Sorghum flour

3 cups cornstarch

Makes 9 cups.

Keep refrigerated.

Banana Bread or Muffins

From Jean Wright of Allegany, New York

3 over-ripe bananas, mashed

2 Tbsp. butter, softened

1 cup sugar

1 egg

2 Tbsp. buttermilk or "sour milk"*

1 tsp. baking soda

1/2 tsp. GF baking powder

1/2 tsp. regular or sea salt

2 cups flour (use GF mixture with 2 tsp. xanthan gum)

1/2 cup walnuts, finely chopped (optional)

1/2 cup raisins (optional)

Preheat oven to 350 degrees F. Grease and flour (with GF flour) loaf pan. Mix ingredients thoroughly. Pour into prepared loaf pan. Bake for 1 hour. For 12 muffins made from the same batter, bake 25 minutes.

*To make sour milk: Place at least 2 Tbsp. milk in a dish and add a few drops of cider vinegar. Let sit 5 minutes until it curdles.

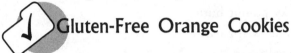

Gluten-Free Orange Cookies

From Barbara Emch of Hubbard, Ohio

Rind and juice of 5 oranges, combined and set aside.

3 cups Bette Hagman's GF mix

1 tsp. xanthan gum

1 tsp. baking soda

2 tsp. GF baking powder

1 1/4 cups sugar

1 cup vegetable shortening

3 eggs

1/4 cup applesauce

Preheat oven at 375 degrees F. In one bowl, mix the dry ingredients. In another bowl, cream the sugar, shortening, eggs, and applesauce. Add 1 cup of juice and rind to creamed mixture. Next, add the dry ingredients to the creamed ingredients and mix well. Drop teaspoonfuls 2 inches apart onto greased baking sheet and bake for 10–15 minutes. Frost with gluten-free orange frosting.

Peanut Butter Christmas Balls*

From Teresa A. Van Nuland of Kenosha, Wisconsin

2 cups GF cereal crushed

2 sticks margarine

1/2 cup chunky peanut butter

2/3 cup coconut, well-packed

3 cups powdered sugar

1 tsp. vanilla

5 Tbsp. butterscotch chips

5 Tbsp. chocolate chips

1/6 stick paraffin (wax found in grocery canning section)

Cream the margarine and peanut butter together. Next add powdered sugar gradually while mixing at low speed to avoid dust. Add coconut, cereal crumbs, and vanilla. Mix well and form into 1 1/4-inch sized balls by hand. Set balls aside.

Melt butterscotch and chocolate chips with paraffin in the microwave. (If this mixture cools, you may need to re-melt for use.) Dip balls to coat, then remove to cool on waxed paper.

Makes approx. 40 balls.

*For this gluten-free adaptation, use EnvironKidz brand "Gorilla Munch," Imperial margarine, Skippy/Jif PB, Baker's flaked coconut, Crystal powdered sugar, and Authentic Foods' brand Premium Vanilla Powder (reduce amount to 1/4 tsp. vanilla powder). For butterscotch and chocolate chips, I use Baker's or Hershey's brand.

Thin Mint Cookies

From Teresa A. Van Nuland of Kenosha, Wisconsin

Tastes just like the Girl Scouts version.

40 unflavored round crackers

1/2 cup chocolate chips

10 drops GF mint or peppermint extract

1/6 stick paraffin (wax found in grocery canning section)

Melt chocolate chips and paraffin together in microwave, stirring occasionally to blend. Add drops of mint extract. Stir. Dip cracker into melted chocolate (using small tongs or fingers to coat). It may be necessary to reheat chocolate/paraffin mixture periodically as it begins to harden. Remove coated cracker and place on wax paper for drying. Store in refrigerator to prevent melting or store at room temperature if desired.

For gluten-free brands, use Bi-Aglut snack crackers, Hershey or Baker's chocolate chips, and McCormick's brand of mint extract.

 ## German Chocolate Cake

From *www.glutenfreeda.com*

Makes one 3-layer cake.

Use the Gluten-Free Pantry's Country French Bread Mix.

2 1/4 cups GF flour

1 tsp. baking soda

1/2 tsp. salt

4 ounces semi-sweet GF chocolate, chopped

1/2 cup boiling water

1 cup crème fraiche

1 tsp. vanilla

1 stick unsalted butter, room temperature

1/2 cup vegetable oil

1 3/4 cups sugar

5 large eggs

Preheat oven to 350 degrees F. Grease and flour three 9-inch cake pans and line the bottoms with parchment paper. In a medium bowl, sift together, flour, baking soda, and salt. Set aside. In a small bowl combine chocolate and boiling water and stir until chocolate is melted. Set aside. In a small bowl add 1 cup crème fraiche and vanilla. Set aside. In a large bowl, beat 1 stick butter and oil on high until lighter in color and texture. Beat in sugar slowly. Beat in 5 egg yolks, one at a time. Add the chocolate and beat just until combined. Alternately, add and beat on low speed, the flour mixture and the crème fraiche. In a separate bowl, beat the egg whites until soft peaks form.

Fold egg white mixture into the batter. Stir gently until combined and pour evenly into the cake pans. Bake for 30 minutes or until an inserted toothpick comes out clean. Let cakes cool on a rack.

For frosting:

1 cup sugar

1 cup crème fraiche

1 stick unsalted butter, cut into small pieces

3 large egg yolks

1 1/3 cups unsweetened coconut

1 1/3 cups pecans, chopped

Combine sugar, crème fraiche, butter, and egg yolks in a small saucepan and bring to a boil. Reduce the heat to low and cook for 1–2 minutes, stirring constantly. Remove from heat and stir in coconut and pecans. Let cool.

Remove one cake from the pan and place on a cake platter, right side up. With a sharp knife, cut the crown of the cake so it is flat and level. Top with 1/3 frosting; do not frost the sides of the cake. Repeat with remaining layers.

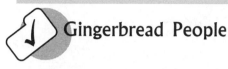 Gingerbread People

From Bonnie J. Kruszka, author of *Eating Gluten-Free with Emily* (Xlibris Publishing, 2003)

1/2 cup shortening

2 1/2 cups Bette's Gourmet Four Flour Blend

1/2 cup sugar

1/2 cup molasses

1 egg

1 Tbsp. vinegar

1 tsp. GF baking powder

1 tsp. ground ginger

1/2 tsp. baking soda

1/2 tsp. cinnamon

1/2 tsp. ground cloves

In mixing bowl beat shortening with an electric mixer on medium speed for 30 seconds. Add about half of the flour, the sugar, molasses, egg, vinegar, baking powder, ginger, baking soda, cinnamon, and cloves. Beat until combined. Beat in remaining flour. Cover and chill for 3 hours or until easy to handle.

Divide the chilled dough in half. On a lightly floured surface, roll half of the dough at a time 1/8-inch thick. Cut desired shapes with a 2-1/2-inch cookie cutter. Place 1 inch apart on a greased cookie sheet. Bake in a 375-degree F. oven for 5 to 6 minutes or until edges are lightly brown. Cool on the cookie sheet for about 1 minute. Remove and cool on wire rack. Makes about 36 cookies.

Chocolate Buttermilk Cake

From Marybeth Doyle of Kirtland Hills, Ohio

3/4 cup oil

2 cups sugar

2 tsp. vanilla

4 eggs

3–4 1-ounce squares baking chocolate

1/2 tsp. xanthan gum

2 cups fern soya powder

1/2 cup potato starch flour

2 tsp. GF baking powder

1 tsp. baking soda

1 1/2 sticks margarine or butter, melted

1 cup milk

Melt the chocolate and let cool. Cream oil, sugar, and vanilla. Add margarine or butter, beat, and then add eggs and beat well. Add the melted chocolate and mix. In a separate bowl, mix flours, xanthan gum, baking powder and backing soda. Add the dry ingredients, alternating with the milk, to the chocolate mixture. Blend well. Pour into greased (use Pam non-stick cooking spray) 11- × 8-inch cake pan. Bake at 350 degrees F. until a knife comes out clean.

Buttermilk frosting:

1/2 cup butter

1/2 cup butter-flavored Crisco

1 tsp. vanilla extract

4 cups powdered sugar

4 Tbsp. mils

Cream together butter and Crisco. Then add vanilla and blend well. Add 1 cup at a time powdered sugar, alternating with 1 Tbsp. milk. Blend well and frost the cooled cake.

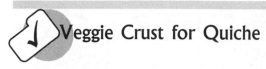

Veggie Crust for Quiche

From Annie Hanaway of Portland, Oregon

1/2 cup grated parsnip

1/2 cup grated zucchini

1/2 tsp. sea salt

1 cup grated carrot

1/3 cup oat flour or mix of walnut meal, quinoa flour corn flour

2 Tbsp. butter, grated

Toss all these together to mix well, and pat into a buttered/greased 9-inch pie pan. Bake at 375 degrees F. for 40 minutes, then cool before filling. The crust will often slide down the sides of the pan a bit during baking so try to put a bit extra on the sides to compensate.

Chapter 7

Gluten-Free for All Occassions

Special occasions, such as parties, weddings, and travel, are a part of everyone's life, whether you have celiac disease or not. Many of these events involve eating food outside of the home and can present new challenges for those on a gluten-free diet. The most important factor is to be prepared for whatever occasion you are about to encounter. Use the knowledge and skills you have learned and follow some of the helpful tips and information in this chapter. Put things in perspective and keep in mind that, no matter what the event is, the actual special occasion, and not the food, is what you are celebrating.

Party On

The key to enjoying parties on your gluten-free diet is to be prepared. One tip is to fill up before you go. It is not a good idea for anyone to get to a party completely famished, but, for the person on a gluten-free diet, it can make things more difficult. Eat before leaving the house when you are headed to a party where there may be limited gluten-free food choices. You can also call the host ahead of time to discuss what will be on the menu. Graciously ask if he or she can put a bowl of salad aside for you before adding croutons and/or salad dressing as well as a plain piece of meat, fish, or chicken before marinade, sauce, or breading is added. Offer to bring a dish or an appetizer so that you know for sure there will be something you can eat. Don't be afraid to ask questions when you eat at a party. Politely ask, "Oh, this looks delicious. What is in it?" And be careful of those utensils that get used for more than one dish or appetizer.

There are all types of great foods that you can serve or bring with you to parties. Adapt some of your favorite party recipes into gluten-free recipes. Good choices include gluten-free birthday cake or other desserts, deviled eggs, gluten-free tortilla chips and gluten-free salsa, sweet and sour gluten-free meatballs, fresh vegetables tray with dip, fresh shrimp, hummus, assorted nuts, stuffed mushrooms, or gluten-free barbecued chicken wings. Use your imagination! (See Chapter 6 for some great recipes.) At the buffet or appetizer table, seek out the fresh vegetables, fresh fruit, and cheese platters. These are usually the safest to eat.

Traveling Tips

No matter how you plan on traveling, be sure to plan ahead. If you are going to fly and your trip is long enough that you will be eating airline food, call the airline at least 24 hours in advance and request a gluten-free meal. There are a number of airlines offering these types of meals.

The following airlines have been known to accommodate passengers that request gluten-free meals in advance:

- Air Canada
- Air New Zealand
- American
- British Airways
- Continental
- Delta
- KLM/Northwest

- Lufthansa
- Qantas
- Swissair
- United Airlines
- US Air
- Virgin Atlantic

This is not an all-inclusive list, so be sure to call the airline you are taking in advance to request information. If you have any doubts about the food that is going to be served, ask if you can bring your own. Even though many airlines now serve gluten-free meals, their understanding of the gluten-free meal may not be up to par. If you order a special meal from the airline and there are breads, muffins, or cookies that have no wrapper, be careful because you won't be able to verify the ingredients. It is best to pack a few snacks to take with you in case your meal isn't quite what you expected.

If you are planning a cruise, compare different cruise lines and find out which ones might be more accommodating to your special dietary needs. Keep a few snacks in your room to eat throughout the day or take with you when you leave the boat for a full-day excursion. Most cruise lines will be accommodating to your dietary needs. Ask about bringing your own mixes for the chef to make up during your stay.

When planning for a car trip, pack a cooler to make sure you have plenty of food for the length of your trip. Pack gluten-free crackers and cheese, peanut butter, gluten-free granola bars, fresh fruit, fresh vegetables, gluten-free cookies, gluten-free candy, or nuts. (Don't forget to pack plenty of water, too!)

When traveling out of the United States double-check the label and ingredient lists on foods that are labeled "gluten-free." Some countries are different in their labeling laws, so be sure you are not being served a product made with wheat starch. In many foreign countries products that are labeled gluten-free may contain up to .3 percent protein (which may possibly be gluten) and wheat starch can be used in their baked goods. Corn flour can be modified food starch on many foreign labels, which means it can contain corn, wheat, or other flour. You can bring some of your own foods on your travel outside the United States, but you may need to have a letter signed by your physician stating it is for medical purposes so that it will not be confiscated.

Research your destination and try to get recommendations about gluten-free friendly restaurants and hotels from local support groups or online message boards. People who live in the area or who have traveled there before can be a big help.

Dining Out

Dining out can be very frustrating for someone with celiac disease. All those choices on the menu that you cannot order! Just as diabetics do, people with food allergies do, or people who are watching their weight do, you must learn to make special choices that do not contain gluten. It is easy to avoid the obvious rolls, pasta, casserole dishes, and breaded meats, but you must look deeper. Has the meat been marinated in some type of sauce before it was cooked? Is the meat floured before it is grilled or broiled? Is the soy sauce made from wheat or soy? Is the rice steamed in water or some type of broth? Were there croutons in the salad that were simply picked out because you ordered it without? What are the ingredients in the salad dressing? It is important to ask questions. Don't be embarrassed to ask the server or even ask to speak to the chef. It is your health and you are paying for your meal! Many celiac organizations now offer "restaurant cards" that give the chef or cook a simple explanation of your special dietary needs. Using a card may help you to feel more comfortable when communicating with the restaurant staff. Make up your own card that you can carry in your purse or wallet for easy access, or check out the following:

- *www.livingwithout.com/diningcards.html*
- *www.triumphdining.com/glutenfreediet.aspx*
- *www.glutenfreepassport.com/traveling/translations.html*

You can also contact your local celiac organization or national organizations about these cards.

Before you dine out, carefully select the restaurant you are going to visit. Choose a restaurant with a large menu selection or restaurants with ethnic foods that are more likely to be gluten-free, such as Mexican, Thai, or Japanese. Avoid buffet-type places where you will not be able to easily find out what is in the foods and how they were prepared. Avoid French and Italian restaurants, where it may be difficult to find a dish that is gluten-free.

Most restaurants (even fast food ones) will offer some type of meal that is gluten-free. Remember everything you have learned about eating gluten-free and verify any questionable ingredients with the staff. If the waitstaff cannot help, ask to speak to the chef or cook. Make sure you not only ask about specific ingredients, but also about food preparation procedures in the kitchen.

Here are some tips to follow when dining out:

- The chef and waitstaff may not be as knowledgeable as you about gluten-free diets, so be specific when asking about certain dishes.

- Explain to the staff that you have a serious food allergy and that their help is greatly appreciated. Even though a food allergy is not what you technically have, most people will respond more quickly to that. Be polite and descriptive about your dilemma, not demanding or difficult.

- Choose restaurants that have foods that are made to order and menu choices that are simple.

- Call the restaurant and talk to the manager or chef ahead of time to be sure they can accommodate your needs.

- Explain cross-contamination and that your meal needs to be prepared using a separate, clean pan and separate, clean utensils.

- Opt for a baked potato as a side dish instead of rice, which is often cooked in chicken stock or bouillon. Stay away from potato dishes that contain additional ingredients or potatoes that are fried (the same oil may be used for other batter-fried foods).

- Order menu items that are simple, such as grilled chicken or broiled fish and ask them to top with fresh lemon, olive oil, or fresh herbs. Make sure it is not floured before being cooked. A basic choice also ensure that the chef is not picking out forbidden ingredients.

- Be sure that your salad does not contain croutons and did not come in contact with them. Bring your own salad dressing so you don't have to worry about checking the ingredients of the restaurants brands.

- Ask servers not to place garnishes on your dish in case they contain gluten.

- When ordering hamburgers, be sure they are 100-percent beef and have no fillers and that the hamburger buns are not toasted on the same grill surfaces where the burgers are cooked.

- Take a look at the appetizer list. There is nothing wrong with potato skins topped with cheese and bacon bits or shrimp cocktail as a meal. Be careful of potato skins and nacho chips that are fried with gluten containing foods. Ask that your skins be baked instead of fried.

- If you feel comfortable, bring your own crackers, bread, or nachos. Some restaurants will allow you to bring in your own bread. Do not send it to the kitchen though; simply order your sandwich without the bread and build it at the table. If you are unsure, call the restaurant ahead of time to ask about their policy.

Terms to Know When Eating Out

Avoid	Ask About	Order
Au gratin	Dressing	Broiled
Bisque	Fried food	Fresh
Breaded	Imitation	Grilled
Coated	Marinated	Pan seared
Casserole	Sauce	Poached
Creamed	Sauté	Roasted
Croutons	Soufflé	Steamed
Processed	Soup	
Roux	Stew	
Stuffing	Stir-fry	

Restaurants to Visit

Many restaurants are beginning to acknowledge gluten-free foods and dishes, so don't be afraid to eat out. Find specific restaurants in your area that you can trust will give you choices and serve you a safe gluten-free meal.

The Gluten-Free Restaurant Awareness Program (GFRAP), whose Website can be found at *http://www.glutenfreerestaurants.org*, can suggest possible restaurants that provide gluten-free meals. Restaurants can choose to participate in the GFRAP, which will aid them in being able to properly provide gluten-free dining.

There are some restaurant chains that do serve gluten-free foods, both fast food and sit-down style restaurants. However, you must still remain vigilant and do your homework before visiting the restaurant of your choice. Keep in mind that just as manufacturer's change recipes, ingredients, and procedures so do restaurants. Therefore, check often to obtain the most up-to-date information. Don't always assume that once gluten-free always gluten-free!

Taco Bell

Taco Bell has stated that because wheat is a part of so many of its recipes, many items served at Taco Bell restaurants are not suitable for gluten-free diets. However, there are a few "Suggestions for Wheat and Gluten Sensitive Individuals" that they state on their Website:

- Tostada
- Chicken Fiesta Taco Salad (order without the shell and without the Red Strips)
- Chicken Express Taco Salad (order Chicken instead of Beef)
- Zesty Chicken Border Bowl (order without the Zesty Dressing and without the Red Strips)
- Southwest Steak Bowl (order without the Creamy Jalapeno Sauce)

Taco Bell has stated that its nacho chips, even though they do not contain wheat, are now fried at each store and are fried in the same fryer in which wheat-containing items are prepared. You can contact Taco Bell at 1(800)-tacobell or visit the Website at *www.tacobell.com* for more information.

Wendy's

Wendy's offers several items that are considered gluten-free. For a full list visit the following page on their Website, *www.wendys.com/food/pdf/us/gluten_free_list.pdf*.

You can request additional information from Wendy's about their menu at:

Consumers Relations Department
Wendy's International, Inc.,
One Dave Thomas Blvd.
Dublin, OH 43017
(614) 764–3100 Ext. 2032
www.wendys.com

Arby´s

Arby's provides a food allergens list on their Website, which does contain information on foods that contain gluten. You can learn more by visiting their Website at *www.arbys.com* or calling 1 (800) 487–2729.

Dairy Queen (DQ)

Dairy Queen lists gluten-free foods on its Website at *www.dairyqueen.com*. The following items are listed as gluten-free:

- Vanilla and chocolate soft serve
- Artic Rush Slush (all flavors)
- Moolatte

(Note: this does not contain hazelnut flavored drinks)

Its supplier of manufactured novelties also states the following are gluten-free:

- DQ Fudge Bar
- DQ Vanilla Orange Bar
- Dilly Bar

There is also a list of Blizzard treats as well as toppings that are safe to eat. Dairy Queen notes to check all of this information with your local restaurant. The corporate number is (952)-830–0200.

Boston Market

Boston Market does list allergens, including gluten, on their Website although they do not guarantee that cross-contamination with gluten-containing foods will not occur.

Boston Market Corporation
14103 Denver West Parkway
Golden, CO 80401
1(800) 365–7000
www.bostonmarket.com

Subway

Subway provides information on many allergens in its foods including wheat and gluten. The list is updated regularly. You should check the Website at *www.subway.com* or call (800) 888–4848 for more information.

Outback Steakhouse

Outback Steakhouse is very accommodating to gluten-free patrons. It has a menu online that can be printed out to inform you of which menu items are gluten-free. To contact Outback Steakhouse, visit *www.outback.com*.

Chipotle Mexican Restaurant

At Chipolte everything is gluten-free except the wheat tortillas for burritos, the soft flour/wheat taco tortillas, and the Hot Red Tomatillo Salsa. The Website does explain that their corn could have a small amount of gluten from cross-contamination with gluten-containing grains in the field. They warn that if you are highly sensitive, you should request that the server change his or her gloves and that they would be happy to do so. They also state that because their employees work with wheat tortillas all day long, there may be the possibility of cross-contamination in our restaurants. Contact Chipotle at *www.chipotle.com*.

Carrabba's Italian Grill

Carrabba's Italian Grill, in cooperation with the Gluten Intolerance Group (GIG) now offers a gluten-free menu. You can find it at *www.carrabbas.com/menu.asp*.

PF Chang's China Bistro

PF Chang's offers a special gluten-free menu upon request. See their menu at *www.pfchangs.com/pdfs/gluten.pdf*.

McDonald's

McDonald's no longer maintains a list of products that are considered gluten-free. They state that they do, however, provide extensive nutrition and ingredient information for all of their nationally offered menu products on their Website (*http://www.mcdonalds.com/usa/eat.html*) and that it is updated frequently, as they receive new information from their product suppliers. They encourage consumers to read their ingredient statements and make personal decisions that best fit their dietary needs.

This is not an all-inclusive list of restaurants that provide gluten-free foods or meals. This is only a sample to prove that you can enjoy dining out even on a gluten-free diet. If you are interested in visiting a particular restaurant, do your research and investigate what it has to offer. Keep in mind that the world of gluten-free foods is becoming much more accepted and recognized, so you may find local restaurants, such as pizza shops, that are now offering gluten-free alternatives. As always, not every restaurant, even chains, will follow the same procedures.

The information provided in this chapter can be updated at any time, so check with companies frequently to be sure menu changes have not been made.

Websites and companies that are great resources for travel and restaurant information include:

- Good Health Publishing, LLC
  (*www.goodhealthpublishing.com/index.html*)
- What? No Wheat? Enterprises
  (*www.whatnowheat.com*)
- CeliacTravel.com (*www.celiactravel.com/index.html*)
- Bob and Ruth's Gluten-free Dining and Travel Club
  (*www.bobandruths.com*)
- InnSeekers (*www.innseekers.com*)

Check with your local celiac organization. Many of them have comprised lists of restaurants in your area that serve gluten-free meals.

Chapter 8

Tips for Living Every Day on a Gluten-Free Diet

The following are tips from people who have celiac disease and live with a gluten-free diet every day. These people are experts in their own right, and their advice is invaluable.

From Regina Celano of Ronkonkoma, New York

- It's a good idea to find out which gluten-free medications you may need based on your health history. For instance, I am prone to sinus infections. Before I went to the doctor, I found out that the antibiotic Levaquin was gluten-free. If you go to the doctor unprepared, you may find yourself diagnosed and then having to do your research afterward. That's a delay of a day or two until you get your prescriptions. Are you prone to ear infections, anxiety attacks, or insomnia? Make a list of gluten-free prescription medications to give to your doctor to keep in your chart and keep a copy at home, too.
- Invest in a soft-sided thermal bag with a shoulder strap and a few of the ice bags you freeze (instead of blocks, which add weight).

163

- Run, don't walk, to your local support group.
- Always, and I mean always, have gluten-free snacks handy in the cabinets and fridge, such as carrot and celery sticks, string cheese, rice crackers, and peanuts.
- Never be without some homemade gluten-free muffins, brownies, or other quick desserts.
- Invest in a good gluten-free cookbook, such as Roben Ryberg's *Gluten-Free Kitchen* (Three Rivers Press, 2000) and Jax Peters Lowell's *Against The Grain* (Henry Holt, 1996).
- The most important staples for the kitchen are Kinnik-Kwik Bread Mix from *www.kinnikinnick.com*, Chebe Bread Mix from *www.chebe.com*, and Gluten-Free Pantry Mixes for sandwich bread, muffins, and brownies from *www.glutenfree.com*; many health-food and grocery stores carry them now. All of these staples have various uses and you can never have enough on hand, so stock up.

From Kit Kellison of Chesapeake, Virginia

- Take your cell phone to the grocery store to call manufacturers about the contents of their foods. State that you have celiac disease and that you get severe damage from eating food with gluten in it, and ask if any gluten is added to their product. Asking whether something is "gluten-free" is not enough; something may have a small amount of gluten and still be considered "gluten-free." Every time you call a manufacturer, it takes up someone's time and costs someone money. This is important because the more time that is spent fielding consumers' phone calls about the allergens in products, the more likely a company will be to address this issue on labels. Remember to be polite and concise during your inquiries. Send e-mails or letters if they don't print their phone numbers on their labels.

- Join the Delphi Forum Celiac Online Support Group (*http://forums.delphiforums.com/celiac*). It has the most up-to-date list of member-verified safe foods, a wonderful gourmet cook who contributes daily, and members who are doctors who have the disease or have children who have the disease. It offers the ability to communicate with hundreds of other people with celiac disease about a range of topics and has been found to be indispensable by many grateful people who have celiac disease.

- Download medical studies to give to all healthcare providers with whom you may come into contact, including dentists who may spot dental enamel defects or doctors of other specialties who can be instrumental in getting someone diagnosed. Two weeks after I brought information to my endocrinologist, she told me about positive serum results for celiac disease on two of her patients. Boy, were their GIs embarrassed!

- Get a good set of knives, and learn how to use them. I often cook from scratch three times a day, so I have gotten nearly as fast as a sous chef when prepping for meals. A good, sharp, heavy, chef knife is easier to control than a little paring knife when cutting the many vegetables and fruits prepared in a gluten-free kitchen. It is much easier to clean one knife than it is to clean all the parts of your food processor.

- Place a standing order at Kinnikinnick Foods (*www.kinnikinnick.com*), which automatically ships my breads, cookies, donuts, and muffins every two weeks so my kids don't have to go without. This also helps my children learn self-discipline; if they aren't careful to eat reasonable portions of goodies, they pay the consequences by having to wait for the next shipment.

- Get rid of, or segregate, all Teflon, dishcloths, wooden spoons, wooden cutting boards, toasters, and iron skillets that were I use before the kitchen became gluten-free. All of these things are porous or absorbent and can contaminate the things a person with celiac disease eats or eats with.

- Use paper towels to clean up in the kitchen so gluten isn't spread to other dishes. Better yet, keep a fully gluten-free kitchen. Everyone will eat healthier, and the gluten-eaters can enjoy their pizzas and hamburgers while out of the house. I had to resort to this strategy when I realized my teenagers were spreading crumbs throughout the house whenever I was not there to monitor their activities. Not surprisingly, I no longer have unexplained bouts of nausea and diarrhea!

- Always keep corn flour, potato flour, or potato starch on hand. I use corn flour for breading because, unlike other gluten-free flours, it will allow the meat to become cooked before the coating burns to a hard, black shell. Potato flour and starch are the best thickeners for soups, sauces, and gravies. A supply of crushed gluten-free cornflakes and gluten-free breadcrumbs in the freezer will make life much easier should you need them.

From Jessica Duvall of Williamsburg, Kansas

- Be a self-advocate. Don't sit by and rely on others to provide you with the information you need. Seek it and you will be empowered.

- When you cook a meal, cook an extra portion to freeze for those times when you need a quick dinner.

- Build a network made up of supportive family, friends, other people with celiac disease, Internet groups, and books.
- Stay strong; you will have good days and bad days.

From Marcy Thorner of New Market, Maryland

- Keep a notebook or computer file of manufacturer contacts. Include their phone numbers and dates of contact for each product. It's a good idea to schedule rechecks periodically on products that you use frequently.

- Check with the host of a children's birthday party to find out what he or she is planning to serve. Send a similar gluten-free item for your child. If you can't stay to help serve and supervise, make special arrangements ahead of time with the host or plan to show up at serving time. Volunteer to provide the ice cream and make it a gluten-free brand. Ask that the host set aside a serving of ice cream in a separate container so as to eliminate the risk of contamination from a serving spoon contacting cake.

- Always send a snack bag with a child who has celiac disease for a play date, and include items that can be shared, such as microwave popcorn, fresh fruit, raisins, and cheese sticks. A child with celiac disease will feel less isolated if his or her snacks are acceptable to playmates.

- Help teach young children with celiac disease to make good food choices very early by labeling pantry and refrigerator items that are gluten-free with a fun sticker. Tell the child, "You can help yourself to the things with the Spiderman sticker, but the others will make you sick."

- Come up with a catchy way to refer to your child's gluten-free foods. If the child's first name is Allison, for example, call it "Special Allison Food" and use the acronym "SAF." Enlist the aid of older children (siblings, playmates, cousins, and so forth) to help supervise at family gatherings or parties. Don't convey a ton of responsibility, but suggest that they come and get you right away if they see your child reaching for the cookies, cake, and so on.

- Keep a gluten-free grill and a separate toaster for gluten-free bread.

- Don't use wooden spoons or cutting boards.

- Enlist the aid of your gluten-free children in determining whether certain foods are acceptable. Start them reading labels very young, and be patient when they struggle with difficult words. Engage children in being proactive, in making good decisions, and in acquiring knowledge about what is healthy for them. Start early to make it a lifelong habit.

- Keep it simple when ordering at restaurants. Mention "celiac disease" by name, just in case the server might be knowledgeable, but don't count on that to communicate your needs. Say, "My daughter (or I) have celiac disease, which is like a food allergy." Most people understand that food allergies can have dire consequences, and that should be adequate to engage them in helping to safeguard your child's health or your health. If not, don't hesitate to ask for the manager or chef.

- If at all possible, call ahead when you are planning to dine out. Let a manager or chef know that you will be needing some special assistance. Tell him or her when you are coming and discuss menu items that may be suitable.

- I like Bette Hagman's flour mixes. I often add a few tablespoons of bean flour and/or cornstarch to the mix (replacing an equal amount). My impression is that the greater number of flours used in a blend, and the less plain rice flour used, the better.

- Look for recipes that use very little flour. I would always select a torte recipe that uses no flour or only a few tablespoons over a regular cake recipe that calls for a couple of cups.

From Miki Ruffino of Destrehan, Louisiana

- I like to keep lots of fresh fruit on hand, washed and ready to eat in sealable bags. Orville Redenbacher Natural Popcorn for the microwave is another handy snack.

- When I first found out I had celiac disease, it was absolutely all I could think about. But time heals that initial shock and then we settle into the everyday routine. It is like any other major change I made. After 21 days it became a habit.

From Lila Brendel of Bismarck, North Dakota

- I put a red sticker on my gluten-free items after I purchase them so my family knows they are gluten-free (for example, the butter, jelly, and peanut butter). Also, after I read labels of common foods and find them gluten-free, I put a sticker on them so I don't have to re-read the ingredients. I also do this if I make a gluten-free casserole with pasta and freeze it. I order pasta, snacks, and flour in large quantities (to save on shipping) and freeze them.

- I always have a container of gluten-free powder cream soup mix and gluten-free pancake mix on hand in the freezer.

- I use tomato juice in place of tomato soup in casseroles and thicken with minute tapioca or Knox gelatin.

From Pat Bridges Welland, ON, Canada

- If you aren't 100-percent sure something is gluten-free, don't eat it.
- I never go anywhere without packing either my small or large cooler (depending on the length of the trip) with nonperishable foods and drinks, including cutlery, serviettes, and cups.
- Don't let other people's negative attitudes get to you. You know what's best. If they can't deal with it, so be it.

From an Anonymous Contributor

- Read labels, re-read labels, and then read labels again. Many companies change ingredients frequently. Know what to look for on your label. Know the key words.
- Always ask questions in restaurants and everyone's home—even your own parents' home, after 50 years.
- Always be polite, grateful, and gracious.
- Think of what you can eat, not what you cannot eat.

From Connie Rieper of Fayetteville, Arkansas

- Don't be afraid to experiment.
- Just as rice cooks at low temperatures, rice flour does cook best at lower oven temperatures (250–300 degrees F.).
- If the outside of your food cooks (or burns) and the inside is wet, then the cooking temperature is too high!

From Jason Estes of Fayetteville, Arkansas

Just because it is meat doesn't mean it is gluten-free. It may have additives, preservatives, and flavorings.

From Wendy Percival of Kansas City, Missouri

- At children's schools, I have kept frozen gluten-free cupcakes in the nurse's freezer, kept a box of gluten-free candy choices in the classroom, or even sent something special when I knew there would be a treat in the classroom.

- At birthday parties I usually ask if I can send along a plate of gluten-free brownies or something so that my kids can share with the other guests as well. If there will be pizza, sometimes we bring our own along or eat before we go. Often, if I explain our circumstances, the hosts are happy to provide a snack my kids can eat.

From Kristine Green of Woodlawn, Tennessee

- I keep my most-used recipes and ingredient lists for mixes on my refrigerator for quick reference.

- I store all flours and starches in the refrigerator or freezer to help them last longer and to save cabinet space.

- I convert short, simple recipes to gluten-free and always look for already-gluten-free recipes.

- For college students, instead of purchasing a food token, book, or card to buy food at the cafeteria, take that money and put it into an account at a bank nearby. Use that account to order gluten-free foods throughout the year. Set it up so that only certain amounts of money can come out as orders and as cash per day. The cash can be used for drinks, fruits, or snacks on campus. This way the money is only used for food, and there are no worries of cross-contamination. If orders are made every so many days, instead of all at once, then storage won't be an issue. There are post offices on most campuses for students, so delivery isn't an issue either.

From Rolf Meyersohn of New York, New York

- Don't feel sorry for yourself! Remember that you can eat *everything* except foods that contain gluten.

- We are finally leaving the Dark Ages of prescribed foods. We can drink Scotch, we can eat pickles, and we don't have to fear blue cheese or gorgonzola. Best of all, we can begin to rely on real scientists and real research, instead of counterphobic threats and dire warnings. I suggest reading Dr. Kasarda's contributions on *www.celiac.com*; and you should certainly subscribe to Gluten Free Living (*www.glutenfreeliving.com*).

- For most dishes, you really don't need a special gluten-free cookbook and can rely on the great basic cookbooks, including Christopher Kimball's *The Cook's Bible* (Little, Brown, and Company, 1996). But of course, for baked goods, you do need special recipes. I bake bread based on recipes from Bette Hagman's *The Gluten-Free Gourmet Bakes Bread* (Holt Paperbacks, 2000) as well as the more recent collection by Karen Robertson, *Cooking Gluten-Free* (Celiac Publishing, 2003).

- When you are in a restaurant, it is probably easier to tell the waiter and chef that you have an allergy, rather then trying to explain the problems of celiac disease. The concept of allergy and the dire consequences of trespassing its restrictions are widely understood.

From Barbara Westmoreland of Hampstead, New Hampshire

- Find a doctor and nutritionist who specialize in celiac disease.

- Get on the Internet. Start with *www.celiac.com* and read about the illness. Go to the support group section and get the number of the group nearest you. Call right away and get yourself a local mentor.

- When starting out, revise the home kitchen. Go through and mark everything as good, bad, or unknown, for which I used green, red, and yellow stickers, respectively. Separate the red from the green. If possible, go strictly gluten-free. It's so much easier knowing that if it's there, it's edible for all.

- Subscribe to the St. John's Celiac Listserv (*CELIAC-subscribe-request@LISTSERV.ICORS.ORG*) and read the e-mails every day. I created a folder in my Yahoo mail system, and I place the messages in the appropriate folder if I want to keep it for reference.

- Attend any and all workshops and conferences on the subject of celiac disease and gluten-free diets. There is so much to learn. The sooner you get the required amount of education, the sooner you'll learn to live well with celiac disease and take the diet in stride.

- Subscribe to celiac newsletters.

- Order some cookbooks and start experimenting. Always plan to make two things on any given day, because when you have one for the garbage and one for you, your celebration of the successful one overrides the disappointment in the other. If you only have one, and it goes to the garbage, you're bound to end up in tears. And remember: Every success you have is one more thing that you can safely eat for the rest

of your life. It's not a today treat. It's a forever food.
Make sure you take good care of the recipe.

- Raise awareness by speaking about celiac disease. Help get this disease out of the closet and into the public eye. Celiac disease is the most under-diagnosed chronic condition in America. There are so many people out there who would become healthy again, if they become aware and can be properly diagnosed.

- When the next person tearfully tells you she/he or theirs have just been diagnosed with celiac disease, give them a hug and a loaf of gluten-free bread. Hold their hand and share your knowledge and positive attitude with them. Take them out to lunch, and go shopping for gluten-free food together. Be their lifeline until they are properly empowered.

From Pingkan Lucas of Munich, Bavaria, Germany

My saving grace was looking toward the east. Many Southeast Asian dishes (Thai, Vietnamese, Indonesian, Malaysian) are gluten-free by nature or are easily made into gluten-free meals. The food is delicious, easy to make, and very healthy, with a variety of vegetables, herbs, and spices. This has made my life and my diet more than bearable.

From Trisha B. Lyons, RD LD, MetroHealth Medical Center, of Cleveland, Ohio

- Before you begin a gluten-free diet for life, please be sure your celiac disease diagnosis was made carefully through thorough medical evaluation.

- Upon your diagnosis, it is important to visit with a dietitian who thoroughly understands celiac disease and the gluten-free diet.

- Inaccurate information abounds where the gluten-free diet is concerned, particularly on the Internet. Please be careful what you read and believe.

From Christine A. Krahling of Easton, Pennsylvania

- Upon diagnosis, it is essential to work with a gastro-enterologist and dietitian who are familiar with the basics of the gluten-free diet and up-to-date on the latest developments concerning celiac disease. Don't hesitate to keep searching until you find the professional that best meets your post-diagnosis needs.

- Try to select professionals who can provide you with basic guidelines for a gluten-free diet and refer you to the national celiac organizations, related Websites, and a support group in your community, if there is one. If there isn't one, think of starting one!

- As you learn the basics of the GF diet, keep a surplus of foods on hand for last minute travel and emergencies such as power outages. These surplus foods can include rice cakes, gluten-free crackers, gelatin desserts, cereals, and pretzels.

From Bonnie J. Kruszka of Newbury, Ohio, author of *Eating Gluten-Free with Emily* (Book Surge, 2009)

Search for a celiac disease support group. You may just find lifelong friends in the process!

From Barbara Emch of Hubbard, Ohio

- The hardest thing to deal with has been going to weddings, reunions, and other special occasions. It is best to call the caterer: Many times he or she can make you a gluten-free version of what the other guests are having. Call in the early afternoon before the chef gets busy.

- Remember that many of your favorite recipes can be made gluten-free, and they are just as good and maybe better. I have successfully done this for almost all my favorite recipes.
- Remember to be positive. People who feel sorry for themselves are tiresome, and they are not helping themselves at all.

From MaryBeth Doyle of Kirtland Hills, Ohio

- Never feel deprived. It will soon become second nature to prepare gluten-free meals.
- Always travel with some gluten-free food, because it is not as readily available as other foods. The airlines never seem to completely understand this diet.
- Designate your own toaster, bread machine, and tub of margarine.
- Clean utensils used for condiments when making gluten-free sandwiches and regular sandwiches at the same time to prevent cross-contamination.

From Kirsten Klinghammer of Rescue, California

- I remember being in the hospital after coming out of surgery and being given my first meal with not one single thing on the tray that I could eat; this was after giving them a detailed list of what was okay and what wasn't! Now, if I need to be checked into the hospital, I just bring my own food and vitamins and have my family bring me more food as needed. I would make sure the doctor okays everything, too.

From Dawn Croft, RD LD of Washington, DC

Be cautious of similar food items made by different manufacturers. Each manufacturer includes its own additives, so just because one brand is gluten-free, doesn't mean they all are.

From Yvonne Gifford and Jessica Hale of *Glutenfreeda.com*

- There are many wonderful recipes that are naturally gluten-free. This eliminates the need to modify recipes and spend time and money searching for hard to find gluten-free products.

- Consider taking advantage of polenta, quinoa, wild rice, and many other delicious, naturally gluten-free products.

- Always keep a well-stocked pantry. Make your own chicken stock by using leftover, unused chicken parts and freeze the stock in one-cup portions for convenience. It not only is better for you, but it tastes better as well.

- To improve your gluten-free baked goods, try adding an extra egg to your recipe and substituting vegetable or canola oil for butter. In addition, when converting your favorite baked goods recipes, choose recipes that have two cups of flour or less.

From Katrina Morales of Tampa, Florida

- Even though there are gluten-free noodles readily available, there are naturally gluten-free products that can easily be used as substitutes, such as using a roll of prepared polenta in place of lasagna noodles. Simply cut it in 1/4-inch slices and layer like you would the noodles.

- Good gluten-free brands include Tinkyada Pasta Joy (*www.tinkyada.com*), Kinnikinnick, Pamela's Baking Mixes (*www.pamelasproducts.com*), Chebe Bread Mixes, and Laura's Gluten Free Rolled Oats (*www.lauraswholesomejunkfood.com*).

- Triumph Dining Cards are invaluable when it comes to eating out. These laminated cards clearly list foods containing gluten, questionable foods, and safe foods. Better yet, these cards are cuisine specific and multi-lingual. All cards are written in both English and the native language of the specific cuisine.

- Restaurants with gluten-free menus include Outback Steakhouse, Maggiano's, PF Chang's, Carrabba's, and Legal Seafood.

- Experimentation is the key to finding products that fit your specific needs and tastes.

From Lauren of Dublin, California

- First and foremost, invest in a bread maker. It will make all the difference. I am *not* a cook and the thought of baking bread from scratch was just too much for me. I bought a bread maker and ordered the Favorite Sandwich Bread from the Gluten-Free Pantry and it changed my life. The bread is tasty and easy to make. It cuts easily and, as the name implies, is great for sandwiches. I will bake a loaf and freeze some of it, so I always have some available.

- There are several muffin mixes on the market. You can purchase these at any health food store, Trader Joe's, Whole Foods, or even your local grocery store. I work for Safeway, Inc., and I'm able to purchase the Sandwich Bread and Muffin mix there. I can find ready-made gluten-free pizza crusts from Whole Foods. I just take one home, add my own toppings, and I'm able to enjoy pizza. I also purchase pasta made with rice flour, and I'm able to enjoy any pasta dish. My family doesn't even know the difference anymore!

- Make sure to ask your local store manager if they carry any gluten-free products. You might be surprised. If not, many grocery stores carry flours that are used for baking, such as rice flour, potato flour, and others.

- When eating out I usually choose Mexican food. It's the easiest food to eat out, as so much of it is corn-based, though you still need to ask questions about how certain restaurants prepare their foods.

- Grilling out is an easy option to avoid having to deal with any gluten. We grill a lot, and it's yummy, healthy, and gluten-free.

- Check if any bakeries in your area will bake gluten-free products. There are a few bakeries where I live that have some gluten-free items. It never hurts to ask.

- Search online for recipes. You can Google "gluten-free recipes" and find almost anything online.

- As a first step, I joined the Celiac Sprue Association (CSA). You can join online (*www.csaceliacs.org*) and there is a wealth of information about celiac disease.

From Jennifer Marrs of Cornish, New Hampshire

- Bring your own packets of salad dressing with you to restaurants. Usually you can at least get a salad (no croutons!) if nothing else on the menu looks safe. The dressing is often the big questionable, so I always bring my own in case the dressing offered is either unknown or contains gluten.

- I often find that fruit comes to the rescue. If I am stuck on the road or end up in a café, I can usually score a banana or an apple. It seems like every gas station, Starbucks, and convenience store in my area has a few pieces of fruit for sale. It is something that I know is safe to eat and it's good for me too!

From Susan of Portland, Oregon

In restaurants, I usually order some sort of meat without the sauce or pasta. Restaurants are noisy and waiters are often young and in a hurry. The best way to really make it clear to them is to ask for "bare naked" chicken or "bare naked" pork. Usually they are embarrassed or they giggle but they do get the idea. Tell them to cook it in a separate pan and specify what oil they can use, if any. And give good tips so they are nice to the next person with allergies or celiac disease who comes in.

From Stacy Baran of Manchester, Maryland

I've only been gluten-free for nine days, but I've noticed such an amazing difference in how I feel. Whenever I want something like real pasta, non-gluten-free beer, or just one bite of the grilled cheese sandwich I made for my 2-year-old, I just remind myself of how far I've come already and how big of a setback that one bite or sip would be. So far, that has kept me completely on track.

From Rob of Princeton, New Jersey

If you don't like to cook, having a slow cooker with a timer has been a life saver. I load it up in the morning and it is ready when I get home.

From Laura D. Huerta of Oakley, California

It used to be a problem when co-workers would invite me to lunch, because they would invariably choose to go to a Japanese restaurant, bad news for a person with celiac disease who is allergic to seafood. I now keep wheat-free tamari sauce in the fridge at work and bring it along to use on the salad and meats. The restaurants never protest. Likewise, when my family wants to eat Mexican food, I bring my own corn tortillas and gluten-free beer.

From Sally Hara, MS, RD, CDE, CSSD of Proactive Nutrition

I would recommend the rice/almond and rice/coconut flours by Gluten Free Mama (*www.glutenfreemama.com*). If the person doesn't have nut allergies or sensitivities, these are great products. I discovered them this year after my mom sent me a cookbook that uses them, and I've been hooked ever since! They have a great consistency and no bitter taste, unlike so many gluten-free flours. After the only local source for these products recently stopped carrying them, I decided to sell them so that they are still available to myself and my patients.

From Annie Hanaway, naturopathic physician, of Portland, Oregon

- I use nut meals often, especially hazelnut, almond, and walnut meal. Pecan is delicious, though I don't use it as much because it's so expensive. These can easily replace wheat germ or small amounts of flour when it's just used for thickening. They add a lovely flavor. You can get them at Trader Joe's.

- I use Bob's Red Mill flours. Most health food stores will carry them. There are some amazing flours—coconut, amaranth, teff, garbanzo/fava—that are excellent for gluten-free baking.

From Stephanie O'Dea (*www.crockpot365.blogspot.com*) of San Francisco, California

I have never been much of a cook. I get side-tracked easily, and often would allow pots to over-boil on the stove, or let items in the oven burn to a crisp. When our family was diagnosed with celiac disease, I knew that I would need to overcome my fear of the kitchen and make most of our family meals by scratch. Instead of enrolling in a crash-course in Cooking 101, I began to cook most of our meals the only way I knew how: I used my Crock-Pot.

Crock-Pots are an invaluable tool for a family with allergies. Fresh or frozen meat can simmer in an inexpensive, gluten-free sauce and be served over brown rice at the end of a long day. Dried beans can be cooked to perfection with little work; and can be frozen for use in future meals.

Our family travels with our Crock-Pot. To ease dinnertime trauma, I will place some stew or chili into the Crock-Pot before leaving for a day of sight-seeing. We arrive "home" to a fully cooked meal that we can eat in our pajamas. This is much more relaxing than trying to navigate a gluten-ridden restaurant menu.

I was blown away at how packaged gluten-free sandwich bread cooked perfectly in the moist environment of a Crock-Pot. There is no rising time needed—just whip up the dough according to manufacturer's instructions and place in a greased round Crock-Pot, or you can put an oven-safe loaf pan directly into a larger oval model. Vent the lid with a chopstick or wooden spoon, and cook on high for 2 1/2 to 5 hours. My bread usually takes about 3 3/4 hours in a 6-quart Crock-Pot. The bread is done when it is brown, pulls away from the pan, and an inserted knife comes out clean.

Chapter 9

Resource Guide

The resource information listed in this chapter is believed to be reliable and correct at the time of the printing of this book. The author assumes no liability for any errors or recent changes in contact information. Some companies produce both gluten-free and gluten-containing foods. Though most manufactures take extra precautions to prevent cross contamination, not all of them guarantee that their products are 100-percent gluten-free. You should question each manufacturer you purchase foods from about its individual guarantee.

The following list is far from being all-inclusive; however, these resources will help get you started and will open the door to discovering even more.

Valuable Information Websites

American Celiac Disease Alliance: *http://americanceliac.org*

Celiac.com: *www.celiac.com*

Celiacs, Inc.: *www.e-celiacs.org*

Clan Thompson Celiac Page: *www.celiacsite.com/index.php3*

Finer Health & Nutrition: *www.finerhealth.com*

Glutenfreeda.com, Inc.: *www.glutenfreeda.com*

Gluten Free Drugs: *www.glutenfreedrugs.com*

Glutenfree.com: *www.glutenfree.com*

Gluten-Free-Online.com: *www.gluten-free-online.com*

The Gluten Free Page—Celiac Disease/Gluten Intolerance Web sites: *http://gflinks.com*

Mayo Clinic: *www.mayoclinic.com*

The North American Society for Pediatric Gastroenterology, Hepatology, and Nutrition (NASPGHAN): *www.naspghan.org*

University of Maryland Center for Celiac Research: *www.celiaccenter.org*

U.S. Department of Health and Human Services/National Institutes of Health: *www.nih.gov*

USDA Nutrient Database for Standard Reference: *www.nal.usda.gov/fnic*

Cookbooks (by Author)

Carol Fenster, Ph.D.

Savory Palate, Inc.

8174 South Holly St., #404

Centennial, CO 80122

(800) 741–5418; (303) 741–5408

E-mail: info@savorypalate.com

www.savorypalate.com

Wheat-Free Recipes & Menus (Avery, 2004)

Cooking Free (Avery, 2005)

Gluten-Free Quick & Easy (Avery, 2007)

Gluten-Free 101 (Savory Palate, 2008)

1,000 Gluten-Free Recipes (Wiley, 2008)

Bette Hagman

The Gluten-Free Gourmet Bakes Bread (Holt Paperbacks, 2000)

The Gluten-Free Gourmet Living Well Without Wheat, Revised Edition (Holt Paperbacks, 2000)

More From the Gluten-Free Gourmet Delicious Dining Without Wheat (Holt Paperbacks, 2000)

The Gluten-Free Gourmet Cooks Fast and Healthy (Holt Paperbacks, 2000)

The Gluten-Free Gourmet Makes Dessert (Holt Paperbacks, 2003)

The Gluten-Free Gourmet Cooks Comfort Foods (Holt Paperbacks, 2004)

Easy Gluten-Free Cooking (John Blake Publishing, 2007)

Karen Robertson

Cooking Gluten Free! A Food Lovers Collection of Chef and Family Recipes Without Gluten or Wheat (Celiac Publishing, 2003)

Roben Ryberg

The Gluten-Free Kitchen: Over 135 Delicious Recipes for People with Gluten Intolerance or Wheat Allergy (Three Rivers Press, 2000)

You Won't Believe It's Gluten-Free!: 500 Delicious, Foolproof Recipes for Healthy Living (Da Capo Press, 2008)

Sheri L. Sanderson

Incredible Edible Gluten-Free Food for Kids (Woodbine House, 2002)

Connie Sarros

E-mail: gfcookbook@hotmail.com

www.gfbooks.homestead.com

Gluten-Free Cooking for Dummies (co-authored with Danna Korn) (For Dummies, 2008)

Wheat-Free Gluten-free Dessert Cookbook (Gluten Free Cookbooks, 2003)

Wheat-free Gluten-free Recipes for Special Diets (Connie Sarros, 2004)

Wheat-free Gluten-free Reduced Calorie Cookbook (Gluten Free Cookbooks, 2003)

Wheat-free Gluten-free Cookbook for Kids and Busy Adults (McGraw-Hill, 2003)

DVD: *All You Wanted To Know About Gluten-free Cooking*

Anne Sheasby

Eating for Health: Gluten-Free Cooking (Hermes House, 2000)

50 Gluten-Free Recipes (Southwater, 2006)

Foodservice Company

Celinal Foods
689 Talamini Road
Bridgewater, NJ 08807
(908) 704-7017
Founder: Ronni Alicea
www.celinalfoods.com

Cooking Schools, Online Menus, Recipe Sites and Shopping Guides

GFree Online Menu Planning Service
Carol Fenster, Ph.D.
www.GFreeCuisine.com

Glutenfreeda Online Cooking Magazine
Glutenfreeda, Inc.
P.O. Box 1364
Glenwood Springs, CO 81602
www.glutenfreeda.com

The Natural Gourmet
48 W. 21st St., 2nd floor
New York, NY 10010
(212) 645–5170
E-mail: info@naturalgourmetschool.com
www.naturalgourmetschool.com

What? No Wheat? Enterprises
4757 E. Greenway Rd., Suite 107B # 91
Phoenix, AZ 85032
E-mail: whatnowheat@whatnowheat.com
www.whatnowheat.com

The Visual Guide
www.thevisualguide.com/glutenfree.htm

Karina's Kitchen
http://glutenfreegoddess.blogspot.com

The Gluten Free Kitchen
http://gfkitchen.server101.com

A Year of Crock-Potting
www.crockpot365.blogspot.com

Shopping Guide for the Gluten-Free Consumer
Grace Johnston
P.O. Box 367
Lewisville, NC 27023
E-mail: jimjgrace@windstream@net

Amazon.com
www.amazongrocery.com

The Gluten-Free Mall
4927 Sonoma Hwy., Ste C1
Santa Rosa, CA 95409
(866) 575-3720
www.glutenfreemall.com

The Essential Gluten-Free Grocery Guide
www.triumphdining.com

Cecilia's Marketplace Gluten-Free Grocery Shopping Guide
www.ceciliasmarketplace.com

Books (by Author)

Shelley Case, BSc, RD
Case Nutrition Consulting, Inc.
www.glutenfreediet.ca
Gluten-Free Diet: A Comprehensive Resource Guide, Revised and Expanded Edition (Case Nutrition Consulting, October 2008)

Danna Korn
www.glutenfreedom.net
Living Gluten Free for Dummies (For Dummies, 2006)
Wheat-Free, Worry-Free (Hay House, 2002)
Kids with Celiac Disease: A Family Guide to Raising Happy, Healthy, Gluten-Free Children (Woodbine House, 2001)

Bonnie J. Kruszka
Eating Gluten-Free with Emily: A Story for Children With Celiac Disease (BookSurge, 2003)

Tricia Thompson, MS, RD
www.glutenfreedietitian.com
The Gluten-Free Nutrition Guide (McGraw-Hill, 2008)
The Complete Idiot's Guide to Gluten-Free Eating (Alpha, 2007)

Associations and Groups

American College of Gastroenterology
P.O. Box 342260
Bethesda, MD 20827
(301) 263-9000
www.acg.gi.org

American Dietetic Association
120 South Riverside Plaza, Suite 2000
Chicago, Illinois 60606-6995
(800) 877–1600
www.eatright.org

Canadian Celiac Association
5170 Dixie Road, Suite 204
Mississauga, ON L4W 1E3 CANADA
(800) 363–7296
E-mail: info@celiac.ca
www.celiac.ca

Celiac Disease Foundation (CDF)
13251 Ventura Boulevard, Suite #1
Studio City, CA 91604
(818) 990–2354
E-mail: cdf@celiac.org
www.celiac.org

Celiac Sprue Association/USA
P.O. Box 31700
Omaha, NE 68131
(877) CSA–4CSA
E-mail: celiacs@csaceliacs.org
www.csaceliacs.org

Gluten Intolerance Group (GIG) of North America
31214 124th Ave SE
Auburn, WA 98092
(253) 833-6655
E-mail: info@gluten.net
www.gluten.net

Traveling and Dining Out

InnSeekers
http://www.innseekers.com

Bob & Ruth's Gluten-free Dining & Travel Club
http://www.bobandruths.com

CeliacTravel.com
www.celiactravel.com/index.html

Triumph Dining
http://www.triumphdining.com

GlutenFree Passport
www.glutenfreepassport.com

Dietitians Specializing in Gluten-Free Diets

Jean Wolcott, RD, CDN
Upstate Cerebral Palsy
1020 Mary Street
Utica, NY 13501
E-mail: jean.wolcott@upstatecp.org

Shelley Case, BSc, RD
Case Nutrition Consulting, Inc.
E-mail: scase@accesscomm.ca
www.glutenfreediet.ca

Theresa Cornelius, MS, RD, LDN, CLT
7424 Oaken Dr.
Knoxville, TN 37938
(865) 922-8780
E-mail: theonlineceliacdietitian@yahoo.com
www.reallivingnutrition.com/TheresaCornelius.aspx
http://nutrition.bitwine.com/advisors/tcorneli
www.changing-lifestyles.com

Melinda Dennis, MS, RD, LDN
Delete the Wheat, LLC
Founder/owner of Delete the Wheat: Nutritional Counseling for the Gluten-Free Diet
E-mail: MelindaRD@deletethewheat.com
www.DeletetheWheat.com

Sally Hara, MS, RD, CDE, CSSD
Registered Dietitian, Certified Diabetes Educator, Board Certified Specialist in Sports Dietetics
ProActive Nutrition, LLC
Kirkland, WA
E-mail: proactivenutrition@msn.com
(425) 814-8443

Cheryl Harris, MPH, RD, LD
Harris Whole Health
3345 Duke St.
Alexandria, VA 22314
(571) 271-8742
E-mail: cheryl@harriswholehealth.com
www.harriswholehealth.com
Personal Blog: *www.gfgoodness.com*

Cindy Hartman, RD
Holistic Chef/Nutrition Education Coordinator
(512) 663-8393
E-mail: ktchndancer@yahoo.com
Michal Hogan, RD, LD, CLT
(866) 396-4438
www.nutritionresults.com

Cynthia Kupper, RD
Executive Director, Gluten Intolerance Group of North America
31214 124th Ave. SE
Auburn, WA 98092
(253) 833-6655, ext. 104
www.gluten.net
www.gfco.org
www.glutenfreerestaurants.org

Trisha B. Lyons, RD, LD
Department of Clinical Nutrition
MetroHealth Medical Center
Cleveland, OH 44109
(216) 778–4952 (for appointments)
E-mail: Tlyons@metrohealth.org

Angela B. Moore, MS, RD, LD/N, CLT
ACSM Certified Exercise Specialist
Certified LEAP Therapist for Food Sensitivities and Intolerances
FitLife of Colorado
(720) 201-1128 (Denver)
(970) 726-2877 (Winter Park/ Fraser)
E-mail: angela@fitlifeofcolorado.com
www.fitlifeofcolorado.com

Carol Rees Parrish, RD, MS
Department of Nutrition Services
University of Virginia Health System
Digestive Health Center of Excellence
Charlottesville, VA 22908
(434) 924–2286
E-mail: crp3a@virginia.edu

Jan Patenaude, RD
Consultant, Writer, Speaker
Director of Medical Nutrition
Signet Diagnostic Corporation
(970) 963-3695
E-mail: DineRight4@aol.com
American Dietetic Association
Find a Nutrition Professional
www.eatright.org
Sub-Group of American Dietetic Association
Medical Nutrition Practice Group
E-mail: sharretm@chi.osu.edu
www.mnpgdpg.org

Support Groups and Online Groups

Raising Our Celiac Kids (R.O.C.K)
National Celiac Disease Support Group
Danna Korn
E-mail: Rock@celiackids.com
www.celiackids.com
Find a support group in your area:
www.enabling.org/ia/celiac/#support

Gluten Free Casein Free Diet (GFCF) Diet Support Group
www.gfcfdiet.com

Delphiforums Celiac Disease Online Support Group
http://forums.delphiforums.com/celiac

Celiac.com Forum
www.glutenfreeforum.com

Celiac Listserv at St Johns University (New York, USA)
E-mail: CELIAC-subscribe-request@LISTSERV.ICORS.ORG

Newsletters and Publications

Celiac.com's Guide to a Scott-Free Life Without Gluten
E-mail: info@celiac.com
www.celiac.com

Gluten-Free Living
Ann Whelan, founder and editor/publisher
P.O. Box 375
Maple Shade, NJ 08052
(800) 324–8781
E-mail: info@glutenfreeliving.com
www.glutenfreeliving.com

Glutenfreeda Online Cooking Magazine
Glutenfreeda, Inc.
P.O. Box 1364
Glenwood Springs, CO 81602
www.glutenfreeda.com

Living Without
800 Connecticut Ave.
Norwalk, CT 06854
www.livingwithout.com

Connie Sarros Gluten-free Newsletter-ette
http://gfbooks.homestead.com

Gluten-Free Food Companies and Distributors

Amy's Kitchen
(707) 578–7270
www.amyskitchen.com

Authentic Foods
(310) 366–7612
E-mail: sales@authenticfoods.com
www.authenticfoods.com

Bob's Red Mill
(800) 553–2258
www.bobsredmill.com

'Cause You're Special! Gourmet Gluten-Free Foods
(866) NO–WHEAT, (866) 669–4328
E-mail: Info@causeyourespecial.com
www.causeyourespecial.com

Chebe Bread Products
1840 Lundberg Drive
Spirit Lake, IA 51360
(800) 217–9510
E-mail: info@chebe.com
www.chebe.com

Dietary Specialties
10 Leslie Court
Whippany, NJ 07981
(888) 640–2800

E-mail: info@dietspec.com
www.dietspec.com

Eden Foods, Inc.
701 Tecumseh Road
Clinton, Michigan 49236
(888) 424–EDEN (3336)
E-mail: info@edenfoods.com
www.edenfoods.com

Ener-G Foods, Inc.
5960 First Avenue South
P.O. Box 84487
Seattle, WA 98124
(800) 331–5222
E-mail: customerservice@ener-g.com
www.ener-g.com

Enjoy Life Foods, LLC
3810 River Road
Schiller Park, IL 60176
(847) 260–0300
www.enjoylifefoods.com

Freeda Vitamins
47-25 34th Street, 3rd Floor
Long Island City, NY 11101
(800) 777–3737
E-mail: info@freedavitamins.com
www.freedavitamins.com

Gluten Evolution
Breads From Anna
(877) 354–3886
E-mail: info@glutenevolution.com
www.glutenevolution.com

Gluten Free & Fabulous
(480) 947–7315
E-mail: info@glutenfreefabulous.com
www.glutenfreefabulous.com

Gluten Free Mama
Gluten Free Mama Kitchen, LLC
P.O. Box 478
Polson, MT 59860
(406) 883–6426
www.glutenfreemama.com

Gourmetfoodmall.com
www.gourmetfoodmall.com

Glutenfree.com
P.O. Box 840
Glastonbury, CT 06033
(800) 291–8386
E-mail: pantry@glutenfree.com
www.glutenfree.com

Gluten-Free Trading Co., LLC
3116 S. Chase Ave.
Milwaukee, WI 53207
(414) 747–8700
E-mail: info@food4celiacs.com
www.gluten-free.net

Gluten Solutions
E-mail: info@glutensolutions.com
www.glutensolutions.com

Glutino Food Group
Canada
(800) 363–3438
E-mail: info@glutino.com
www.glutino.com

Kingsmill Foods
(416) 755–1124
E-mail: kingsmill@kingsmillfoods.com
www.kingsmillfoods.com

Kinnikinnick Foods
Canada
(877) 503–4466
E-mail: info@kinnikinnick.com
www.kinnikinnick.ca

Laurel's Sweet Treats
(866) 225–3432
E-mail: Sales@GlutenFreeMixes.com
www.glutenfreemixes.com

Pamela's Products
www.pamelasproducts.com

Road's End Organics, Inc.
www.roadsendorganics.com

Tinkyada Rice Pasta
Food Directions, Inc.
www.tinkyada.com

Trader Joe's
www.traderjoes.com

Twin Valley Mills, LLC
RR 1 Box 45
Ruskin, NE 68974
(402) 279–3965
E-mail: sorghumflour@hotmail.com
www.twinvalleymills.com

Whole Foods Market
www.wholefoodsmarket.com

Index